Advanced Practice Nursing Ethics in Chronic Disease Self-Management

Barbara Redman, PhD, MBE, FAAN, has been dean of the Wayne State University College of Nursing since 1998. An internationally respected researcher and author in the field of bioethics and a highly regarded administrator and teacher, she formerly served as dean of nursing at both the University of Connecticut and the University of Colorado. Dean Redman has also been executive director of the American Nurses Association and the American Association of Colleges of Nursing. She holds doctoral and master's degrees from the University of Minnesota, a master's degree in bioethics from the University of Pennyslvania, and a bachelor's degree in nursing from South Dakota State University.

Advanced Practice Nursing Ethics in Chronic Disease Self-Management

Barbara Klug Redman, PhD, MBE, FAAN

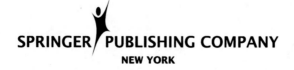

SPRINGER PUBLISHING COMPANY

NEW YORK

Copyright © 2013 Springer Publishing Company, LLC

Springer Publishing Company, LLC
11 West 42nd Street
New York, NY 10036
www.springerpub.com

Acquisitions Editor: Allan Graubard
Composition: diacriTech

ISBN: 978-0-8261-9572-2
E-book ISBN: 978-0-8261-9573-9

12 13 14 15/5 4 3 2 1

The author and the publisher of this Work have made every effort to use sources believed to be reliable to provide information that is accurate and compatible with the standards generally accepted at the time of publication. Because medical science is continually advancing, our knowledge base continues to expand. Therefore, as new information becomes available, changes in procedures become necessary. We recommend that the reader always consult current research and specific institutional policies before performing any clinical procedure. The author and publisher shall not be liable for any special, consequential, or exemplary damages resulting, in whole or in part, from the readers' use of, or reliance on, the information contained in this book. The publisher has no responsibility for the persistence or accuracy of URLs for external or third-party Internet Web sites referred to in this publication and does not guarantee that any content on such Web sites is, or will remain, accurate or appropriate.

Library of Congress Cataloging-in-Publication Data
Redman, Barbara Klug.
  Advanced practice nursing ethics in chronic disease self-management/Barbara Klug Redman.
    p. cm.
  Includes bibliographical references and index.
  ISBN 978-0-8261-9572-2 — ISBN 978-0-8261-9573-9 (ebook) 1. Patient education. 2. Self-care, Health. 3. Chronic diseases—Treatment. I. Title.
  R727.4.R424 2013
  613—dc23
                                        2012021176

Special discounts on bulk quantities of our books are available to corporations, professional associations, pharmaceutical companies, health care organizations, and other qualifying groups.

If you are interested in a custom book, including chapters from more than one of our titles, we can provide that service as well.

For details, please contact:
Special Sales Department, Springer Publishing Company, LLC
11 West 42nd Street, 15th Floor, New York, NY 10036-8002
Phone: 877-687-7476 or 212-431-4370; Fax: 212-941-7842
Email: sales@springerpub.com

Printed in the United States of America by Gasch Printing.

Contents

Abbreviations

ADE	adverse drug event
ADHD	attention-deficit/hyperactivity disorder
AF	atrial fibrillation
BGSM or SMBG	blood glucose self-management
BP	blood pressure
CCM	Chronic Care Model
CD	compact disc
CHW	community health workers
CKD	chronic kidney disease
CMS	Center for Medicare and Medicaid Services
COPD	chronic obstructive pulmonary disease
CTI	care transitions intervention
DSN	diabetes specialist nurse
DVD	digital video disc
ECG	electrocardiogram
EBM	evidence-based medicine
GAS	goal attainment scaling
HbA1C	hemoglobin A1C
HCV	hepatitis C
INR	international normalized rate
MI	motivational interviewing

NHS	United Kingdom's National Health Service
OMERACT	outcome measures in rheumatology clinical trials
P4P	pay for performance
PCORI	Patient-Centered Outcomes Research Institute
PHR	personal health records
PSM or **SM**	patient self-management
RA	rheumatoid arthritis
RCT	randomized controlled trial
SDM	shared decision making
SE	self-efficacy
TA	technology assessment
UTI	urinary tract infection
VA	Veterans Administration

Preface

Patient self-management (PSM) is defined as an individual's capability to detect and manage the symptoms, treatment, physical and psychosocial consequences, and lifestyle changes (e.g., exercise and diet) inherent in living with a chronic disease (Barlow, Wright, Sheasby, Turner, & Hainsworth, 2002). Many acute illness episodes and treatment plans in health care are in fact but one phase in the course of a chronic condition. Efficacy of health care depends on addressing these happenings within an individual's plan for long-term chronic disease management.

PSM has arisen to prominence as part of a broader concept of patient education for two reasons: (1) governments in many developed countries believe they must manage the ballooning costs of chronic disease in their aging populations by shifting care responsibilities to patients and their families, and (2) the patient empowerment movement stresses that a person makes care choices from available options and is free to incorporate these selections into his values and lifestyle. The freedom to choose care options is a growing philosophy in some countries and in others a legal right, instigating the move to PSM.

The reorientation of health care toward PSM invites us to reconceptualize basic assumptions that have been problematic in patient education theory and practice. For example, a great deal of confusion cascades from our failure to consider the appropriate ends of PSM as well as its support. A common misperception is that the proper outcome of PSM is adherence with the prescribed medical regimen and its support must operate under the physician's authority. At an obvious level, this provider-focused assumption denies the patient any say in the regimen and assumes (often incorrectly) that providers follow whatever standard of care is relevant for the patient. More significantly, this framework denies the patient the explicit goal of developing his own practice of PSM that is consistent with both his instrumental goals and the intrinsic value of education.

A second misperception follows from the first; that a dose of patient education at the time of diagnosis is sufficient for support of PSM of chronic diseases. In truth, support must continue across a lifetime to accommodate changes in the patient's body and psychosocial situation and to incorporate new scientific findings. The decisions patients are asked to make as part of PSM are clinically and cognitively (and frequently emotionally) complex. Research has focused on patient deficits in learning the complex skills required for PSM, when, in reality, its mastery should be expected to take considerable time as patients build increasingly sophisticated skills.

Underlying both these misperceptions is one even more basic. Statistically, nearly all individuals will have one or more chronic diseases as they age. (This is not to deny that children also have chronic disease.) Whether currently recognized or not, the fact is that all chronic diseases require PSM. Yet support services are widely unavailable to those who need them, even in countries where public policy indicates patients have a right to this support. The rhetoric of patient empowerment, an extremely important value base for PSM, often masks a transfer of responsibility to patients and families beyond their competency to handle care (Redman, 2007). While this proclaiming of values without really delivering their implementation is a common situation in policy, when it occurs it further victimizes patients who need the services, labeling them as the problem.

PSM is a fascinating movement that arouses perspectives on ethics, psychology, technology, and social policy, and one that requires nursing leadership. Advance practice nurses already care for patients with chronic diseases in varying stages and manifestations, including acute exacerbations and multi-morbidity. Yet PSM in health care is firmly stuck in an outdated medical model that, studies show, nurses find ethically problematic. The purpose of this book is to present a framework for a more just and equitable practice of PSM of chronic disease, including its preparation and support, and one that is congruent with a nursing philosophy of practice.

The book is organized as follows. Chapter 1 describes a philosophical approach using capability theory, especially that of Martha Nussbaum. This chapter also addresses other central ethical questions, such as the level of parity that can be reached with PSM—in itself, a question of equity. Also addressed are standard ethical questions about patient choice and safety, appropriate balance of benefit/harm, and standards of practice (currently very rudimentary). In their regard, I suggest a more ethically appropriate model for use.

Chapter 2 summarizes current best practice for supporting PSM of common chronic diseases while Chapter 3 describes intervention strategies that help patients build the capabilities outlined in Chapter 1. These chapters provide a foundation for subsequent chapters that focus on issues that influence advance nursing practice and that have been viewed as problematic, suggesting an ethical resolution congruent with safe practice and the capabilities framework.

Chapter 4 addresses the changes in self (beliefs, motivations, and identity) that accompany effective PSM. Rarely do we consider what we are asking the patient to achieve from psychological, sociocultural, and moral perspectives, including the conflicts that inevitably arise between the patient's "old" and "new" identities, as he or she obtains competency, or not, as self-manager.

Chapters 5 and 6 engage the ethical impact of technologies, including the often implicit perspectives incorporated into measurement instruments, both singly and across the totality of instruments available in the field, and the informational and equipment technologies used in PSM. Both chapters describe the huge amount of work that remains to be done. A stock of morally sufficient and well-validated measurement instruments does not now exist; yet without this infrastructure, the field cannot move forward. Instruments embody values and standards essential to making clinical and social judgments. Because an ethical analysis of the emerging technologies that make PSM possible is very rare, the impacts of these technologies after adoption are frequently problematic.

In some health fields PSM is manifested as part of a total revolution in the philosophy of care. Chapter 7 describes these shifting boundaries. The patient recovery movement in mental health is the best example of a normative shift. In other fields of practice, the boundaries between provider management and PSM are being dramatically pushed. Here, physician-directed self-monitoring of left atrial pressure in persons with advanced chronic heart failure, which can more adequately titrate drugs to the actual physiological condition of the heart (Ritzema et al., 2010), is an apt example. We must bear in mind, though, that other groups of patients present with symptoms that are never diagnosed or with a prolonged diagnostic phase and uncertain treatment plans. These patients often desperately need guidance in the ability to self-manage their symptoms, and all need an approach that encompasses the life span of the disorder, including its acute phases.

Chapter 8 describes how the transition to PSM of chronic disease might transpire and proposes a structure to correct its very uneven development, at least up till now. Obviously, some of the tasks entailed must be political: Setting revised expectations for capability development and choice; naming the tools that can implement these political decisions; and a push for the necessary health care system change.

Any social movement, major new technology, or emerging change in health care practice requires examination of the ethical assumptions on which the trend is based and ongoing dialogue on how the course of its development will enhance human well-being. This book is one such step for accomplishing PSM of chronic disease. To engage the reader in the kind of reflection needed to play an authoritative leadership role in making PSM a reality for those with chronic disease(s), study questions conclude each chapter. And to assist the health care professional in documenting and improving the quality of PSM in the practice setting, the appendices present four instruments with an analysis of their psychometric characteristics as well as additional study questions and ethics definitions.

It is important to note that the book draws on extant research, much of which comes from countries other than the United States. The United Kingdom has most comprehensively adopted PSM as health policy, and the Scandinavian countries reflect patient empowerment as social policy.

Literature from these countries greatly enriches our understanding of how PSM can be developed philosophically and practically.

1

A Suggested Ethical Framework for Patient Self-Management of Chronic Disease

Statistically, chronic disease is the norm in human health events, yet it has long had a negative connotation in the public mind, linked to perceptions of "old" and "sick." In a fully examined practice of patient self-management (PSM), this denigration can change to more positive perceptions and opportunities for growth and control. For this purpose, we need to turn beyond medicine.

PSM has the potential to meet several important ethical precepts that apply to chronic disease, such as: (1) if we can benefit someone without harming anyone else we ought to do so, (2) dignity of human life involves the freedom to live as one wishes, and (3) it is wrong to discriminate against the uneducated or the poor, who suffer more from chronic disease and its effects. To fully implement PSM, these precepts require policies that ensure patient choice, safety, an appropriate benefit/harm balance, and standards of practice for both patients and providers. Currently, however, we lack a framework to unite these precepts and their necessary policies. The usual ethical theories are less than helpful. Utilitarians (who value the aggregate good) don't adequately recognize needs of individuals and ignore the fact that preferences are affected by traditions of oppression (Charlesworth, 2000). Deontologic schools of thought prescribe duties without describing a way to actualize those duties. Communitarians (who believe communities decide what is right and good) have not, in general, addressed the issue of PSM; local societies typically see preferred options as those put forth by the medical community, whose theory of practice does not embrace education of patients.

THE CAPABILITY APPROACH

The capability approach provides a good fit for PSM. It is a broad normative framework for assessment of individual well-being and social arrangements and the design of policies and proposals for social change (Robeyns, 2005). The approach focuses on developing what people are able to do or be, guaranteeing at the least a threshold level necessary for truly human functioning. Nussbaum (2000) asserts that capabilities can be the object of an overlapping consensus among people who have very different conceptions of the good. Of the ten central human capabilities described by Nussbaum, *life* (being able to live to the end of a human life of normal length, not dying prematurely), *bodily health* (being able to have good health), and *practical reason* (being able to form a conception of the good and to engage in critical reflection about the planning of one's life) are the most relevant to health. These and other central capabilities are not mere instruments for human existence, but are understood to have intrinsic value and are vital to making possible any choice of a way of life.

Capabilities offer people the freedom and opportunity to choose and realize certain functionings. For health care, this is a radical framework because it calls for providing all individuals and groups with the capabilities to achieve a self-determined threshold of functioning. In education, that threshold is the level of development beyond which learning is purposeful and can be sustained by the learner. Because learning is an indispensable means through which individuals and groups can improve their lives, capability deprivation is a state that calls for remediation, whereas capability enhancement requires ongoing development (Young, 2009). Sadly, current health care data do not contain adequate information to allow us to conclude what capability sets people have or could develop.

The capability framework is based on the sense that certain human abilities exert a moral claim for development (Nussbaum, 2000). In contrast, to conceive of people as helpless and without agency is to denigrate them and to fail to respect their dignity. It is important to recognize that human capacities require support from the larger society in order for the person to exercise them. Respect for others mandates creating the conditions in which capacities can develop, unfold themselves, and support choice. In fact capacity, not functioning, is the appropriate political goal for all functional aspects of living, including health (Nussbaum, 2009). Sen (2009) notes that there are remediable injustices that can be addressed in the real world with the use of a capability framework. These include women who live in oppressive circumstances but who would, under a capability approach, be guaranteed threshold level of skills to keep themselves and their families healthy to live longer lives. A capability approach would also ensure recognition of those with stigmatizing chronic diseases, for social support and skills that could help avoid health disparities with other populations that can occur with stigma.

The ideals inherent in the capability framework raise questions of how the approach could be operationalized in a fully examined practice of PSM. To address a first concern, collective and family capabilities are clearly important since they can protect vulnerable individuals who have limited capacities as well as protecting persons longitudinally through subsequent generations. However, a holistic view of family is rarely incorporated in a medical approach to PSM. A second concern is that some health care systems have proclaimed PSM a desirable, perhaps even mandatory, approach to treatment without installing appropriate professional support services, a situation that likely increases the caregiving burden, which historically has fallen predominantly on women, beyond its already high level.

A third issue regarding operationalization is whether we should spend the resources to build PSM capabilities in people even though they may choose not to use them, given that freedom of choice is a central tenet of the capability framework. But perhaps the most difficult questions are whether a capability approach to PSM could adequately address the many poor individuals and families with chronic diseases and whether a package of capability development programs included in health care could, in fact, reverse poverty or prevent it.

Clearly, such comprehensive programs would require significant investment to develop not only the instrumental skills but also the social recognition essential to self-confidence and self-respect. The strength of the capability approach is that it accommodates variability in individuals' capacities and their abilities to convert resources into life functionings; its weakness is that priority-setting in the public sphere remains a problem. Chronic illness is both associated with poverty and a cause of it, for without the skills to control the illness and its symptoms, individuals become unable to work or go to school.

In spite of significant advantages of the capability approach to management of chronic disease, patient adherence to the medical plan of care is currently the most common framework used (Redman, 2009). The problem with this approach is that it admits of no patient choice in determining a plan of care that is acceptable to the patient and incorporate the patient's life goals. In addition, the adherence framework operates under two mis-assumptions: first, that the physician's performance meets the standard of care (often not the case) and is worthy of adherence, and second, that lack of adherence (a behavior frequently associated with poverty) is grounds for excluding patients from treatments that are in short supply (e.g., organs for transplant).

Some PSM supporters have embraced a framework of patient empowerment (interventions to generate hope, confidence, and encouragement) to help people with chronic disease gain control of their lives. Meta-analyses using the empowerment approach through education, support groups, and consultation showed improvements in hemoglobin A1c and reduction in cholesterol in persons with diabetes as well as improvements in patient knowledge and quality of life (Joanna Briggs Institute, 2009). Others have described patient empowerment as a process designed to facilitate self-directed behavior change, with the aim of increasing the capacity of patients to think critically and make autonomous, informed decisions. In many empowerment-based education programs, content is presented based on questions and concerns raised by participants. Patients are in charge of determining which decisions they wish to make themselves and which they prefer health professionals to make (Anderson & Funnell, 2010).

But the empowerment approach contains inherent weaknesses. In the first place, it assumes that patients know what they want, but more seriously it does not commit to development of a guaranteed set of capabilities that patients can choose to use. In addition, while patient empowerment would appear finally to have redressed the imbalance of power between physicians and patients, the reforms necessary to employ this approach also represent a political technique of governing, seeking to manage the problem of rising costs by entrenching health care in a market sphere. This means that patients are "empowered" to care for themselves for the primary purpose of saving money in the market for health services. Thus patients are not emancipated but have traded traditional dependency on the medical profession for dependency on the market. In the British National Health Service (NHS), government can deflect political criticism of its management by passing responsibility onto patients and the choices they made (Veitch, 2010). As with the adherence approach, patient capability to allow functioning is not guaranteed.

The empowerment framework in health care and other sectors is part of a neo-liberal political philosophy of citizenship (particularly as analyzed in the context of the United Kingdom) to "liberate" citizens from the state. It seeks to empower citizens by expanding their reach of choice and voice, accompanied by the responsibility to produce the conditions of one's own independence. A critical analysis of this approach reveals the assumption that bad choices result from irresponsible people, as opposed to questioning the "structural distribution of resources, capabilities, and opportunities." Its language of activation and empowerment can mask the dynamic of abandonment (Clarke, 2005). For these reasons a framework of empowerment for PSM of chronic disease must be carefully applied, with clear empirical evidence that it does not in actuality leave patients worse off. In thinking of available frameworks, however, the capability approach appears the best fit for the goals of PSM.

Several salient points can be made about the capability approach. First, it is open to a range of possibilities of individual lifestyle, although it doesn't address the roles of groups and social structures. It does address a common confusion that financial poverty coincides with poverty of functionings; in truth, a paucity of functionings can't always be solved with money. Third, because most available databases in any sector of life do not contain information about people's capability sets, we must define and assess them on our own. Social norms and power relationships, which have solidified in the health care sector, may restrict people's capability sets by normalizing those with less formal education as less capable. Finally, the capability framework can coexist with other frameworks such as empowerment and even partially with that of patient compliance if research supports its importance and patients negotiate goals of compliance.

Perhaps most importantly, the capability approach urges us to stop seeing patients as burdens who don't know how to manage their chronic illnesses and instead understand what capabilities they have and how they want to develop them toward our mutual goals. But we have a second challenge. To a large extent the kind and range of opportunities that allow us to live a life we value depends on what institutions exist and how effectively they operate. Oppressive social structures preclude the building of capabilities (Alexander, 2010). To reflect, how would you rate the health care structures you know in their support or oppression of patients and their struggles to become capable in managing their health?

GOALS FOR PSM OF CHRONIC DISEASE

The underlying goals of the capability approach are protecting, restoring, and promoting the well-being of individuals. Similarly, goals for PSM of chronic disease focus on development of capability/agency to manage a regimen that incorporates personal and medical goals, including management of symptoms, effect of the disease on lifestyle, and maintenance of a sense of self and agency. These skills accumulate over a lifetime.

In thinking of patient goals and the link to development of agency, it is ethically relevant to understand how chronic disease has been framed. Despite the fact that it is now the leading cause of death and disability worldwide and by 2030 will cause more than three-fourths of all deaths, a series of pervasive myths persist that have the effect of blaming the victim or suggesting that nothing can be done. For example, many still believe that through choice of unhealthy lifestyles chronic diseases are self-inflicted, and/or because these are often diseases of aging, public resources would be wasted on those who have achieved a normal lifespan. In fact, chronic health conditions often originate in poverty, disproportionately affect the poor, and are exacerbated by inadequate education, social exclusion, long-lasting psychological stress, and poor access to weak health systems and poor environments (Geneau et al., 2010).

Coinciding with blaming the patient, chronic illnesses have largely been seen through a medical perspective and classified as diseases, which privileges professional expertise in defining what is relevant. The focus on oversight and monitoring of biomarkers by professionals is still dominant, although other indicators such as symptom management and quality of life have become more common. Considerably underdeveloped is an understanding of genuine patient expertise as patients learn through informed strategic experimentation to identify their own unique disease activity markers and find ways to minimize the extent to which disease management characterizes their everyday life (Thorne, 2008).

The current focus on evidence-based medicine (EBM), although touted in policy and practice as all-encompassing, is in fact quite limited in addressing the ethical questions about PSM of chronic disease raised in the preceding. While EBM should be instructive about patient efficacy, the currently available evidence is largely limited to studies of middle-class individuals followed for only one year and which excluded the aged with multiple chronic diseases, thus ignoring social and environmental causes of chronic illness. The effects of the broad social reorganization of chronic illness work to target the individual to serve the government's purpose of decreasing demand on health services is virtually ignored. The Expert Patient Programme in England, implemented by the National Health Service (Rogers, Bury, & Kennedy, 2009), has been hampered not only by the limited research base on PSM efficacy but also by lack of systematic evaluation of the impact of this policy on patients and their family caregivers.

All three current sets of logic—those who have chronic disease have caused it, following medical protocols is prime, and the evidence base is insufficient to undergird broad social policy—form excuses for not setting realistic goals to help patients learn the skills to manage their chronic illnesses.

CONCERNS FOR EQUITY AND PROTECTION OF PATIENT SAFETY

Because it contributes to the range of exercisable or effective opportunities open to us, health is of special moral importance. Failure to protect those opportunities when we could reasonably do so is unjust. We have an obligation to promote normal functioning and to distribute health resources equitably by properly designing social institutions and policies (Daniels, 2008). Development of skills important to successful PSM—capability for decision making, facility to absorb and act on health information often expressed in probabilities, self-confidence in information seeking—is doable. Still, some aspects of the PSM capabilities approach are clearly under-developed in the United States.

The threshold to which capability development is guaranteed is a political decision in each society. In the United States, serious health inequalities raise significant questions about inequities (morally problematic inequalities). Clinical practice guidelines for some chronic diseases such as diabetes, asthma, and hypertension include PSM education but do not commit to a level of capability development or to guaranteed financial coverage of such development for the population. Data found in financial coverage note that 40% of persons with diabetes and 15% of those with asthma get some exposure to education about their condition, which says little about their ability to safely practice PSM (*Healthy People 2010*).

In the United States most decisions about which health care services to reimburse are made by insurers (through benefits packages) who are heavily influenced by what services physicians want to offer. Although PSM of chronic disease has rarely been included in health care coverage, there is no convincing argument why it should not. A relevant question to ask is, does PSM offer more or less value than other services in which currently the patient or provider is reimbursed, such as psychiatric care or other services with an insufficient evidence base? In other words, are like services being treated as like and unlike services as unlike? Considerations of equity presuppose explicit bases for relevant comparisons, which may include: (a) patient demand for the service, (b) cost-effectiveness in the short and long term on medical criteria such as morbidity and mortality, and (c) contribution to life-long capabilities to manage one's health and its disruption.

As we ascertain from this situation, PSM is built on psychological theories such as social cognitive theory but doesn't include the context of socioeconomic factors that exacerbate poor capability development and poor management of chronic disease. For example, low-income populations exposed to low-cost, nutritionally poor foods are particularly vulnerable to chronic disease. Adults with severe levels of food insecurity have more than twice the risk of diabetes and poorer glycemic control than do adult who have ready access to healthful foods (Seligman & Schillinger, 2010).

The health gradient by education is larger for chronic disease than for acute illness precisely because it is possible to learn how to manage chronic conditions (Cutler & Lleras-Muney, 2010). While it is undeniable that formal education level is associated with better health, the moral questions to ask are the degree to which those without that asset can still learn to adequately manage their chronic diseases and what resources are needed to assist the process, weighed against the psychological, social and economic costs of not acting in this direction. What is an appropriate level of equity in PSM of chronic disease?

PSM has lacked serious incorporation of the science of patient safety—witness the dearth of clear practice standards to which practitioners are held accountable, the primitive development and use of robust measurement tools for the range of valued outcomes, and inattention to harms from PSM and/or to the program of preparation for it. This situation is exacerbated by serious quality deficiencies in the medical management of chronic diseases; a recent study found that 30% of costs for six chronic illnesses are expended on services labeled as potentially avoidable complications (PACs). It is estimated that PAC rates might be reduced by 50% for congestive heart failure and coronary artery disease, 40% for diabetes, 60% for chronic obstructive pulmonary disease (COPD) and asthma, and 75% for hypertension (deBrantes, Rastogi, & Painter, 2010).

In the health literature, many trials do not report harms at all, or they report them in a fragmented or suboptimal way, or they do not account for patient withdrawal owing to harms, and trials in some interventions (psychotherapies) almost never report harms (Ioannidis, 2009). This largely seems to be the case in PSM (Albano, Crozet, & d'Ivernois, 2008), although a summary of meta-analyses on the effectiveness of therapeutic patient education in chronic diseases and obesity (only some of which was likely PSM) showed 6% reported worsening of measured outcomes in the education group (Lagger, Pataky, & Golay, 2010). More directly, a medical record review of 111 diabetes patients with limited literacy in an automated phone health IT self-management (SM) program found 111 adverse events and 153 potential adverse events, 93% of which were preventable or ameliorable. Primary care providers were aware of only 13% of incidents and 60% of prevalent (ongoing) events. Diabetes is a communication-sensitive disease, requiring patient and provider collaboration to optimize SM and avoid complications. On the whole, little is known about patient safety in the ambulatory setting, where ongoing care of individuals with chronic disease is carried out (Sarkar et al., 2008).

Indeed, the process of preparing for and supporting PSM may hold risks as well as benefits. As one example, Rogers et al. (2009) report on the inevitable social comparisons among patients in SM skills training programs (many of whom are middle class), which may have the unintended consequence of lowering expectations and help-seeking activities among those in most need, including those from marginalized and lower socioeconomic groups. People are not always successful in resisting the negative emotional consequences of unwanted comparisons, therefore harming their presentation of self as morally worthy and deserving of care (Rogers et al., 2009). In addition, PSM training programs may not check for and correct common learning problems such as confusion or inability to integrate complex material, leaving patients with less self-confidence than they exhibited before the training program. The fact that harms are rarely detected or made legitimate in PSM initiatives can lead to lack of symptom control and poor disease outcomes as well as the unfortunate dynamic of blaming the patient or the family caregiver for not attaining good outcomes.

This lack of oversight in PSM training exists in the face of over-whelming evidence. For example, a meta-analysis of 35 studies totaling 7,413 patients with heart failure showed that only half of such patients received a complete set of instructions at discharge, much less evidence that they were able to act on such instructions (Boren, Wakefield, Gunlock, & Wakefield, 2009). And a meta-analysis of 47 randomized controlled trials (RCTs) that included 7,677 participants with type 2 diabetes showed that PSM interventions had a positive effect (Minet, Moller, Vach, Wagner, & Henriksen, 2010). While these reviews did not summarize results by socioeconomic status, other work shows clearly that the "education gradient"—the enormous differences in life expectancy by education—is true for every demographic group and is present across countries. Studies show that 30% of the education gradient can be accounted for by access to material resources such as gyms and smoking cessation methods, but 10% is due to explicit factual knowledge and 20% to general cognitive ability to acquire, evaluate, and act on information and feel confident in doing so (Cutler & Lleras-Muney, 2010; Pampel, Krueger, & Denney, 2010).

The capability approach addresses both issues of autonomy and justice (everyone should have an opportunity to reach capability to a politically defined minimum level) but doesn't explicitly address the issue of how PSM, as an innovation, should be diffused in a just way. Buchanan, Cole, and Keohane (2011) address the issue of justice in the diffusion of innovations in general, with a frame that sheds light on important issues in PSM. The shortage of PSM education and support reflects a choice our society has made. Innovations like this create opportunity for promoting justice as well as undermining justice if it is not diffused widely (e.g., checked by domination and exclusion). And the fact that important innovations are not occurring can be a concern of justice. From this perspective, forms of PSM undertaken or that could be undertaken by disadvantaged groups must be seriously studied.

Most theories of justice converge on the belief that extreme deprivation is presumptively unjust, and surely so when it is undeserved and unchosen (Allen, 2011). Clearly, then, individuals who don't have access to the support, skills, and materials to safely manage their chronic diseases suffer an injustice. By their nature, most chronic illnesses cannot be dealt with safely without PSM—diabetes must be managed on an hourly and daily basis; asthma and COPD can be managed more intermittently but take on crisis proportion in an exacerbation.

AN ETHICALLY APPROPRIATE MODEL FOR
PSM OF CHRONIC DISEASE

Current health systems contain many correctable flaws for PSM of chronic disease. It has been noted that the United States does not have a system for dealing with chronic illness, which means that efforts toward PSM of these conditions will be vulnerable to failure. The dual focus on PSM as compliance with a medical regimen and dependent on EBM should be nested within a much broader framework of capabilities development and the examination of ethical issues not addressed by EBM. Denigration of individuals as causing their own chronic diseases and being too old for investment and dismissal of the social and economic contributions to their situation serve to blame the victim. By avoiding commitment to explicit goals such as levels of capability and functioning, an empowerment ideology, and the move by governments to transfer responsibility for chronic disease care to the citizen can leave patients and their families responsible for care but without the skills for safety.

In the United States, current data show that few individuals with chronic disease get any exposure to education about how to care for themselves, much less a commitment to long-term coaching to develop capacities that will support PSM functioning. Insurance rarely covers such services, but without any rationale that covered services are more compelling. It is likely that even in countries with a more supportive health policy, implementation of PSM support is very incomplete.

Those committed to the PSM movement, philosophically or by government mandate, must recognize that significant work still remains. The present research base to test adequacy of PSM skills and the interventions needed to develop and sustain them must be greatly expanded to other populations and expanded longitudinally through families, and must furthermore acknowledge and correct harms as well as document benefits.

At the very least, an expanded PSM has the potential to increase patient safety and satisfaction, but to do this it must be patient-centered, caregiver-centered, and voluntary. Patient/caregiver choice in PSM should be accompanied by negotiation of treatment goals and measurement of current knowledge and skills, as well as an assessment of the socioeconomic situation. A "trial of (PSM) therapy" is appropriate.

Subsequent to initial skills development, patients/caregivers must be guaranteed access to coaching by health professionals for the length of their disease, whether in person or by telephone and/or electronic communication. To support safe practice, patients/caregivers and providers should agree to report (with no consequences) evidence of poor practice in prescribing and implementing PSM, as judged against a range of benefits and harms. The resulting data can be used to put in place a program to increase the benefits and correct the harms. Such systematic data, aggregated over groups of individuals, have never existed and are important for discussions about an appropriate balance of benefits and harms from PSM practice. For example, at some point, after multiple trials, PSM may be considered effective or futile for a particular patient/caregiver at that time.

It is important to note that countries' health policies vary widely in support of a defined level of equity, with the United States at the lowest level of this continuum among developed nations. Inequalities kill opportunity and create poverty, and our current haphazard system of offering or not offering PSM, or requiring it without support, is frequently not based on standardized measures of patient skills with good predictive validity, but on provider biases or insurance coverage protocols, neither of which is transparent.

REFLECTIONS ON CAPABILITY FRAMEWORK FOR PSM OF CHRONIC DISEASE

A capability framework (related to human rights) acknowledges that freedom is a good in its own right but also an instrument for attaining other ends (health). As a perspective, it counteracts increasing domination of the market perspective in health care and long-standing pressure from medicine to demand that patients do what physicians tell them to do. It challenges the continuing assumption that allocation of more funds to high tech health procedures will yield more well-being. The capability approaches takes us back to our roots of caring for people in our community, many times in partnership with patients and families. To illustrate, think of public health nurses in urban slums in the early twentieth century who effected change through patient education. Today, individual practitioners and groups can be a force for this positive change, which will nonetheless also require institutional reform.

All plans of life presuppose at least certain core health capabilities. But some have seen a conflict between the implied liberty in the capabilities approach and the freedom to make choices to realize multiple kinds of valued existences and actions as well as how certain choices may affect the health of others. Allen (2011) asserts that these two values (freedom and health) can be seen as co-equal. Liberty is best interpreted in terms of its priority rather than as an absolute claim to noninterference and is democratically contestable.

This tension is best demonstrated in public health policies that target chronic disease control by monitoring lab values (such as HbA1c among persons with diabetes) and notifying patients and providers when values are high. While seen by some as interference in a private matter (particularly when choice to receive the monitoring is variant), a first inclination is to view such out-of-bounds lab surveillance as poor provider practice, lack of SM preparation and support to the patient, or even as a reasoned judgment on the part of both provider and patient that "normal" lab value is not possible or wise for this patient. As seen by this scenario, public health attention to chronic diseases will continue and escalate, reflecting its prominence as the major disease threat today. Occasionally, tension between values of freedom and health as a particular individual sees it will occur.

Ethical analysis, well-reasoned and informed by data when applicable, should be employed to provide clarification to the current system including the emerging PSM movement. We are yet in the early stages of such an analysis. While capability theory clearly expresses a commitment to social justice, gender equality, and a vision of human dignity, it doesn't specifically address historical and structural roots of inequality and the institutional transformation necessary to ameliorate these (Feldman & Gellert, 2006). Subsequent chapters develop important elements of all of these concerns.

SUMMARY

A capability framework offers a better approach to the practice of PSM, with significant advantage over the current medical focus on patient compliance and even over an empowerment approach. Chronic illness, which is statistically very common, offers opportunity for positive growth and dignity in health care. Ethical analysis offers a tool for understanding how to avoid being punitive to those with chronic disease, focusing instead on an obligation to improve safety and equity in a health care system with serious issues in both of these realms.

STUDY QUESTIONS AND ANSWERS

1. What are the central purposes for PSM of chronic disease that benefit both individuals and society?

   Answer: Several objectives can be fulfilled, such as: (1) better quality of life and ability to function, (2) saving resources, (3) better disease management including prevention of exacerbations and slowing of progression, and (4) self-making by incorporating disease management into life goals.

2. Any field of practice requires conceptual and ethical tools. Arguably, those are underdeveloped for PSM of chronic disease. What tools does the capability framework provide and what tools remain to be developed?

   Answer: Most importantly, the capability framework provides an end goal which meets ethical criteria of good for patients and for society. By doing so, it ties health care to the same criteria as other societal aims, such as economic development and social justice, and removes it from the narrow authority of medicine. The capability framework is very short on details—for example for PSM we could ask what capabilities should be developed to allow which functionings, what is a justifiable boundary for patient authority/choice, and how does one get a society to set its limit for resources to be used for this project, justifying its level with other societal goods.

3. What research questions does the capability framework raise beyond those that are currently asked in the field?

   Answer: A number of research questions emerge, such as (a) what are the variety of ways people choose to use their capabilities to SM their chronic diseases, (b) to what extent do capabilities developed for health extend into other areas of life and improve them, and (c) what rationales do societies use when required to explicitly set and justify the minimal level of guaranteed capabilities for health?

4. Some countries have a stated public policy advancing patient empowerment. How useful is this as an ethical/policy base for PSM of chronic disease?

   Answer: Its value in support of development of patient agency is clear. But as a policy it lacks two things—a content goal (empowerment toward what?) and an implementing structure/strategy to force the transition from a provider-focused health system to a more patient-centered health system.

5. How would you assess the following proclamation: "It is morally essential for the health care system to facilitate patient learning"?

   Answer: Patient learning should be assessed against an end goal of human flourishing, and this would be supported by most philosophies that undergird our sense of what is ethical, including the moral framework outlined in this chapter. Perhaps the most important part of an analysis might be to question how our health care system got so far from this moral ideal, and perhaps an answer would be because it focused on a sense of entitlements among health professionals, slighting the welfare of patients.

6. The capabilities approach acknowledges a state of adaptive preference, a view that people's stated preferences can be deformed because they have adapted to an oppressive culture (which they have deeply internalized) and know no other way. Is adaptive preference operating in management of chronic illness?

   Answer: Yes, evidence of it can be seen in the views that the doctor is always right, that patients have no right to choose PSM or receive support for it that makes their care safer or their lives more livable. Adaptive preference can't be identified as unjust or wrongly hierarchical without an overarching framework like the capabilities approach, and furthermore it can't be fixed by information alone (Nussbaum, 2011).

7. Within the capabilities framework there is a huge moral difference between a policy that promotes health and one that promotes health capabilities. What is this moral difference and how does it relate to PSM?

   Answer: Nussbaum (2011) notes that only a policy that promotes health capabilities honors the person's lifestyle choices. As a foundation for PSM, the capabilities approach is quite distant from the current focus on adherence to a medical regimen, which does not admit to respecting patient choice.

8. Health is one of six essential dimensions of well-being, as is self-determination. In their theory of social justice, Faden and Powers (2011) indicate that institutions have two foci: (1) improvement of

well-being, in this case health, and (2) responsibility to combat adverse effects on well-being caused by patterns of systematic disadvantage that can profoundly compromise health. On these terms, how important is being able to manage one's chronic disease(s)?

Answer: The better control PSM can bring to the person's and family's ability to function and exert some control over the disease, as well as the confidence to maintain direction over one's life, can be profound, although not the same for everyone. This theory of social justice fits well with Nussbaum's capabilities approach. The unresolved question is the degree to which the health care system, in conjunction with other social institutions, commits to avoiding or dealing with systematic disadvantage among patients. Currently, some health care systems have more or less unjust access embedded in racism and poverty (Faden & Powers, 2011). Nussbaum's answer is that society must commit to a threshold capability for each individual.

9. How is patient education different from PSM, and is the capability framework relevant as well for patient education?

Answer: While consensus definitions for patient education and for PSM don't exist, I believe those practices exist on a continuum. Patient education is more commonly used for a health issue that is likely to be resolved in one episode, such as an appendectomy, but of course the patient continues to learn SM skills in wound healing, ambulation, etc. PSM is more commonly used in long-term (chronic) health conditions (although surgery may be part of a long term condition) and thus focuses on day-to-day disease management and symptom control and psychosocial and lifestyle adjustment over the long term.

2

State of the Science and Best Self-Management Practices by Disease

> Chronic illness is embedded in the local flow of moral experience, in the struggles of individuals to craft a moral life, and in the aspiration for ethical values that extend beyond a local world and that speak to questions of fairness, justice, doing good in the world and the largely unmarked yet deeply pro-social value of caregiving. (Kleinman & Hall-Clifford, 2010)

From our knowledge of health statistics worldwide, it is clear that management of chronic disease is a global problem and a costly one, with international organizations such as the United Nations creating a global health agenda to address the concern. The overall burden of chronic diseases continues to grow; it is estimated that by 2030 these illnesses will be responsible for 7 in 10 deaths worldwide, with the heaviest burden felt in less affluent nations (Partridge, Mayer-Davis, Sacco, & Balch, 2011). Chronic illnesses are defined as conditions that last a year or more and require ongoing medical attention and/or limit activities of daily living (Parekh, Goodman, Gordon, Koh, & HHS Interagency Workgroup on Chronic Conditions, 2011).

As the quote at the beginning this chapter indicates, the experience of chronic illness is a moral experience as well as a psychological and social passage. National and local policy has largely ignored the entrenched social, economic, and political conditions that shape people's vulnerability and management of disease. Indeed, a dominant narrative for chronic disease is one of negative behavior, the result of sedentary lifestyles and excess of diet and smoking, a logic that privileges diagnostic categories. The disease becomes entangled in the narrative context of people's work, family, and personal life as the patient experiences periods of adequate function and periods of frailty. Thus, families and individuals must restructure routines and self-identities to accommodate the disease and its management. The patient doesn't have the option of being passive (Kleinman & Hall-Clifford, 2010).

In order to define the kinds of capabilities patients must develop to self-manage, we need to understand the kinds of clinical judgments and life adjustments patients can choose as the disease persists. Some are generic to chronic disease and some specific to the disruptions a particular chronic disease or sets of diseases (multi-morbidities) and their known treatments may cause in a patient's life. While patient self-management (PSM) has been defined as "the ability to detect and manage the symptoms and treatment, physical and psychological consequences and lifestyle change inherent in living with chronic conditions" (Barlow, Wright, Sheasby, Turner, & Hainsworth, 2002, p. 178), a more accurate understanding is that particular patients at particular times are capable of self-management (SM) somewhere on a continuum. It is important to note that normative boundaries of responsible SM have not explicitly been defined, but exist implicitly, revealed in constant demands for patient compliance with the medically supported treatment regimen.

Redefinition of this boundary in a manner congruent with current views on patient agency and empowerment is crucial. Perhaps we can roughly define responsible PSM in terms of inclusive goals, such as actions that meet the patient's life goals in partnership with legally and ethically acceptable professional practice. In this framework, examples outside boundaries of acceptable PSM practice include providers who do not allow safe patient experimentation to reach life goals or patients who abuse this experimentation with clearly harmful practices.

So that we may explore the means to a responsible practice of PSM, this chapter outlines capabilities necessary for PSM of common chronic diseases and any ethical analyses that have been done in the field, covering the following illnesses: arthritis and musculoskeletal diseases, asthma and other respiratory diseases, cancer, diabetes, and cardiovascular diseases.

ARTHRITIS AND MUSCULOSKELETAL DISEASES

Musculoskeletal problems including arthritis are highly prevalent, occurring twice as often as heart and circulatory problems, and they are frequently episodic and persistent. Consistent evidence shows that SM programs for osteoarthritis are effective in addressing pain and daily function, but effect sizes from these studies are small. The exercise component has the strongest evidence in its favor and should be considered a key component of PSM of osteoarthritis (May, 2010).

Diagnoses of musculoskeletal problems frequently include osteoarthritis and rheumatoid arthritis and fibromyalgia. Symptom control, particularly of chronic pain and often of fatigue, is a dominant concern and treatment approach. Yet for patients dealing with these illnesses, becoming an effective self-manager is a process and struggle as individuals try to maintain their pre-pain identity while ultimately requiring acceptance of a changing identity. Along the road to diagnosis, patients frequently describe feeling discredited by health care providers and their suffering minimized. Due to this perception, many patients try everything to identify and treat the source of their pain. Fortuitously, initial acceptance of the chronicity of their illness allows individuals to begin testing different ways of managing their conditions and gaining confidence. Yet it also requires becoming knowledgeable about their condition, sometimes with little guidance from the medical community in doing so. While the journey likely needs to occur for successful implementation of PSM, several points of intervention along the route that would assist the patient become obvious (LaChapelle, Lavoie, & Boudreau, 2008).

As well as the primary illness, common comorbidities, especially for rheumatoid arthritis (RA), must also be addressed in PSM of musculoskeletal disease. Depression has been included in PSM programs and as an outcome measure, but cardiovascular disease, which accounts for about half of the excess mortality in RA, is rarely addressed. Although not common, RA or its medications, as well as recently implicated factors such as systemic inflammation, may adversely affect cardiovascular disease risk factors such as hypertension, dyslipidemia, and physical inactivity. In this context, patients' limitation of physical activity due to fear of joint damage must be addressed with reassurance that exercise will not only decrease RA-related inflammation and improve function and mobility without damaging joints but will improve cardiovascular risk as well. Some patients have suggested cardiovascular disease SM should be introduced once control of RA is established (John, Carroll, & Kitas, 2011).

Many people with RA are active at a level considered too low to maintain good health, and physically inactive people with RA have significantly worse cardiovascular risk compared with those who are active. An important aspect of PSM support is addressing this issue. As will be described in greater detail in Chapter 4, patient beliefs (in this case that physical activity can be helpful for managing disease) are highly predictive of whether patients undertake activity. Therefore, routine use of brief measures of patient beliefs and testing of interventions (Ehrlich-Jones et al., 2011) that are factual and persuasive, as well as building patient self-efficacy that exercise will help, are all essential.

Fascinating as well are the various cognitive frames in which diseases and their symptoms are placed. Very common in musculoskeletal disorders, pain is a powerful motivating force that guides treatment-seeking behavior in patients. Most educational programs for this population have used anatomic and biomechanical models for addressing pain, focusing on tissue injury; these programs have shown varying efficacy. An alternative framing of the problem focuses on teaching patients the neurobiology and neurophysiology of pain and pain processing by the nervous system, reconceptualizing their pain as the nervous system interpretation of the threat of the injury rather than an accurate measure of the degree of injury to the tissue. Patients are taught that the nervous system has the ability to increase or decrease its sensitivity/neuroplasticity to help them cope with persistent pain (Louw, Diener, Butler, & Puentedura, 2011).

Studies of this approach have shown a decrease in patient fear and an increase in pain thresholds. Musculoskeletal pain frequently lacks "objective" radiographic correlates (Louw et al., 2011). The question is whether different cognitive approaches (pain may be caused by neural sensitivity rather than by tissue injury; Louw et al., 2011) more helpful to patients in self-managing their pain; further studies are needed.

ASTHMA AND CHRONIC RESPIRATORY DISEASES

Asthma affects nearly 10% of the U.S. population. Asthma symptom control remains poor among sufferers of this chronic illness, and many asthmatics lack awareness of the severity of their disease and the extent of airway obstruction. For decades, asthma treatments have focused on targeting inflammation and relaxing smooth muscles, although prolonged use of long-acting beta-agonists can increase risk of severe exacerbations, and systematic use of steroids can suppress immunity and increase risk of hyperglycemia and diabetes. In up to 10% of patients symptoms are not controlled with any available therapies, and because development of new drugs to address their needs has a high risk of failure, its progress is slow (Webb, 2011).

Although asthma SM education is a key component in international guidelines, this learning is frequently not supported in the United States. Still, extensive clinical research has found that some asthma SM strategies such as written action plans, symptom recognition, and medication and peak flow meter education are effective in improving outcomes (Estes, 2011). Written asthma action plans should include instructions for handling exacerbations such as self-administration of medication, recommendations for identification and long-term control of medications, and avoidance of triggers (Sadof & Kaslovsky, 2011).

A summary of nineteen studies suggests one reason why action plans have been persistently under-used—a mismatch between provider and patient asthma beliefs and experiences. Patients/caregivers perceived asthma as a "variable" condition with intermittent episodes of stability and periods of acute exacerbation requiring treatment. Health professionals regarded it as a long-term condition requiring constant prevention and compliance with medical instructions no matter the patient's experience level, and focused on pharmacological measures and responding to deteriorating asthma. The answer, of course, is to jointly negotiate and merge the models (Ring et al., 2011).

Well-controlled asthma indicates the following markers: daytime symptoms fewer than twice a week, nighttime awakenings fewer than twice a month, no disturbance of exercise tolerance, use of short-acting beta-agonists for symptoms less than twice a week, and one or fewer emergency department visits for asthma or courses of oral steroids for exacerbations in the last six months. Patients will often say their asthma is controlled even when daily symptoms are evident (Sadof & Kaslovsky, 2011). Of the asthma population, 5% to 20% has severe asthma, but a recent study found 22% of these individuals achieved adequate control following assessment and correction of asthma SM skills in a special clinic. Still, as treatment escalates in severe asthma, these individuals become increasingly at risk of inhaler device polypharmacy and therefore inadequate inhaler device technique (McDonald, Vertigan, & Gibson, 2011).

A study of why poor SM may occur among a group of adolescents suggests the need for intervention strategies in which provider and patient share an explanatory model and utilize current information. Some of the adolescents studied were confused about differences between controller and rescue medications or viewed all patterns of controller use as consistent with "control" of their asthma. Many confused quiescent periods and temporary absence of worsening symptoms after reducing or stopping controller medications as indications that they had outgrown their asthma. In addition, the study found chaotic life situations play a role in poor SM (Wamboldt, Bender, & Rankin, 2011), as do low familial expectations of asthma control and patient worries about the safety of daily asthma medications (Sadof & Kaslovsky, 2011).

Because asthma is prevalent in school-age children, programs to identify symptoms and teach SM skills to students and their families have a rich history. At present only one-third of schools have nurses, so case finding is hampered as is family access to care, particularly for minority children of low socioeconomic status. Nonetheless, nationally sponsored school-based programs have been found efficacious; these focus on preventing, recognizing, and managing asthma symptoms (Bruzzese, Evans, & Kattan, 2009).

In the clinical setting, measurement instruments for PSM of asthma are poor. A review of 18 measures of asthma knowledge found none with information about responsiveness to intervention and interpretability (Pink, Pink, & Elwyn, 2009).

Another chronic respiratory illness, chronic obstructive pulmonary disease (COPD), is characterized by airflow limitation that is not fully reversible. Worsening symptoms (exacerbations) may hasten disease progression, yet these symptoms frequently remain unreported and thus not treated, and these patients show higher mortality than do patients without an exacerbation. SM skills should include early detection and taking appropriate action to manage symptoms. As in asthma, one potentially effective SM tool is an action plan, which encourages patients to identify daily variations in symptoms. Data on the effectiveness of action plans for SM of COPD are few; those that do exist show that a written action plan enhances early detection and prompt action, and thus benefits recovery time. However, action plans have not been found to affect the exacerbation rate (Trappenburg et al., 2011). Still, self-treatments incorporated in a SM program for COPD were found to result in fewer exacerbation days at a lower cost while not leading to overtreatment (Effing, Kerstjens, van der Valk, Zielhuis, & van der Palen, 2009).

CANCER

In spite of its often dire character, some individuals have managed cancer as a chronic illness, extending from early detection to survivorship. A review of studies and model programs in cancer PSM may be found in McCorkle et al. (2011). When cancer chemotherapy and radiotherapy treatments remain safe enough to deliver on an outpatient basis, patients learn to participate in their care and manage treatment effects between visits. Beyond this stage, SM for acute care involves understanding signs and symptoms of disease recurrence and managing late-term effects of cancer and cancer treatment. Unfortunately, expectations for patients and families to manage on their own have outpaced development of effective PSM interventions, resulting in an urgent need to translate findings of effective SM strategies into clinical practice (McCorkle et al., 2011).

In addition to the dearth of clinical support for SM of cancer, evidence-based symptom management in oncology care is far from a mature science. Among the most commonly studied symptoms are pain, depression, fatigue, and insomnia; yet, efforts to educate SM of these symptoms remain suboptimal, and few studies have examined the effect of managing multiple symptoms that may co-occur. Lack of consensus on criteria to define symptom experience, including what constitutes a response and what constitutes meaningful changes in symptoms over the course of illness (Given, 2010), surely complicate development of effective PSM intervention.

The above predicaments are unacceptable because intervention points familiar to other chronic diseases also occur with cancer. For example, the way patients autonomously manage their oral chemotherapy was found linked to their beliefs about treatment efficacy and toxicity. Physicians sometimes minimized or hid information on secondary effects of oral chemo during initiation of treatment to encourage better program adherence and control patients' emotions and anxiety. But patients perceived secondary effects as positive and interpreted them as a sign of treatment efficacy, and did not disclose them for fear their physician would reduce the dosage, thus reducing treatment efficacy (Regnier-Denois, Rousset-Guarato, Nourissat, Bourmaud, & Chauvin, 2009). These erroneous beliefs must be dealt with, and unethical and unsafe practices curtailed. To avoid miscommunication, patients need to develop skills in detecting what to do in the event of toxicity from oral chemotherapy.

In fact, improved patient reporting of adverse drug events (ADEs)/ adverse drug reactions is essential in any setting in which patients receive therapy. Studies have shown that cancer patients do not always express their concerns about drug therapy unless their providers ask the specific questions. Many ADEs resulting in hospitalization stemmed from counteractions to medications used to treat comorbidities, such as anticoagulants and anti-hypertensives. Thus, screening for potential problems is also helpful. But because cancer patients often receive chemotherapy with a substantial risk of side effects that may alter drug pharmacokinetics, patients will remain at risk (Miranda et al., 2011). PSM support should develop patient skills in how to identify ADEs and obtain help when needed. Unfortunately, the model in oncology departments still largely conceives of the patient as "captive" to their disease, which, of course is no longer true (Regnier-Denois et al., 2009).

Perhaps because persons with cancer often finish treatment, programs also have been conceived as oriented to "survivorship." Some clinicians believe the survivor period starts with diagnosis, others after completion of active therapy and when the patient is in remission. Survivorship programs may be disease-specific or include all diseases, and they may be community-based and shared between oncology health professionals and primary care providers. They deal with late effects of cancer treatment, surveillance and prevention, management of co-morbid conditions exacerbated by cancer treatment, and lifestyle and psychosocial issues (Gage et al., 2011). Goals for patients appear implied in these programs.

Other times, calls for posttreatment programs focusing on psycho-logical problems such as fear about cancer spreading, uncertainty about the future, and lack of energy are framed as rehabilitation. For example, approximately a year after finishing medical treatment, patients with breast cancer were found to have a substantial need for help with specific problems related to cancer and its treatment (Schmid-Buchi, Halfens, Dassen, & van den Borne, 2011).

At any transition—shifts from one phase of the cancer journey to another—PSM may become particularly challenging. Women with advanced breast cancer identified transitional shifts in their physical, emotional, and social well-being, as for instance when the cancer pro-gressed and there was a need to change therapy. At these times, patient preferences for disease management should be revisited, covering areas such as how to obtain information about the cancer trajectory and other aspects; symptom management; change in identity, roles and relation-ships; and readiness to self-manage. Although SM skills can be used to anticipate and negotiate transitions as they arise, very little research has addressed these issues (Schulman-Green et al., 2011).

CARDIOVASCULAR DISEASES

SM of risk factors such as hypertension and disease treatments such as anticoagulation exemplifies PSM opportunities in cardiovascular disease. Patient management of heart failure is reviewed in Chapter 6 in the context of finely developed measurement instruments. But in general, close moni-toring by both the patient and provider is essential to detect deterioration in cardiovascular function. The monitoring must be scheduled for patients both close to and remote from health care providers and in a manner that engages the patient and teaches SM skills.

Two ways to accomplish this are structured telephone support, which entails provider monitoring, and/or PSM support delivered via telephone, or telemonitoring, which includes transmission of physiologic data, SM education, and medication administration. More advanced telemonitor-ing systems will provide direction about when and how patients can adjust medications themselves and when they need professional support. Both telephone support and telemonitoring can produce a substantial decrease in risk of heart failure hospitalizations; furthermore, telemoni-toring has been found to yield a substantial decrease in all-cause mortality. Other improvement areas linked to telemonitoring include prescribing, patient knowledge, and SM and functional class. The precise mechanisms by which these interventions produce these effects are unclear. There also is a dearth of evidence about how long patients should be supported by these systems (Ingles, Clark, McAlister, Stewart, & Cleland, 2011).

For persons with heart failure, the optimal dose and duration of training is unclear. Medicare has adopted discharge education as a core quality measure that assesses whether patients admitted for heart failure are discharged home with written instructions or educational material. This endeavor likely does not reach the education level needed to improve heart failure outcomes. Baker et al. (2011) tested a "teach-to-goal" support program for use of adjusted-dose diuretics, employing five to eight telephone follow-ups over a month, and found it more effective than a single education session, including for people with low literacy. Teach-to-goal (through repetition and reinforcement) is a well-established strategy in the educational world.

Very specific elements of SM support for patients with heart failure are now being investigated. These patients experience a number of ADEs such as dizziness and nausea, which affect their willingness to take medications and their quality of life. Management of these ADEs appears suboptimal. Patients with an ADE reported significantly more disease-related symptoms in comparison with patients without an ADE and had more negative beliefs about their illness and medications including a strong belief in medication overuse. Patients with heart failure have difficulty differentiating disease and drug-related symptoms. Nurse practitioners could play an important role in educating patients about ADEs and helping them differentiate ADEs from disease symptoms and checking patients' interpretation of symptoms. This is especially important for those who have negative medication beliefs. These are important SM skills for the patients to develop (DeSmedt, Denig, van der Meer, Haaijer-Ruskamp, & Jaarsma, 2011).

Barriers to PSM of cardiovascular disease are seen in current treatment of persons with hypertension, which relies heavily on clinic measurement of blood pressure at one time even though there is a well-documented mean 8.6 mm Hg difference between home and clinic systolic blood pressure as well as within-patient variability over short periods of time. From these clinical measures patients are categorized as having blood pressure that is in or out of control, especially in patients closest to treatment thresholds, and medication is prescribed. As clear indication of the need for SM of hypertension, more frequent clinic measurement would not eliminate the "white-coat effect" on blood pressure readings in this setting. Major organizations have issued position statements supporting use and reimbursement for home blood pressure monitoring and question whether high quality care can be provided without this SM (Powers et al., 2011).

Another cardiovascular illness treatment, anticoagulation, is currently performed in the United States through clinics, even though in European countries PSM of anticoagulation has been linked to patients spending more time in the therapeutic range. This indicates clinic management is not as effective as PSM; furthermore, it is also more wasteful because one cannot predict when a given patient is going to require a change in warfarin dose, thus problematizing frequency of follow-up visits. Future optimizing of anticoagulation PSM should require not only patient self-testing but also online automated management, which gathers and evaluates information from patients and provides instructions to them, alerts the clinician to need for intervention, and documents a virtual visit (10 minutes of clinician time). Medicare now provides reimbursement for self-testing, including more affordable rates if in-person clinic visits can be avoided (Bussey, 2011).

DIABETES

Diabetes affects nearly 8% of Americans, yet fewer than 30% of sufferers appear fully capable of self-managing their disease (Fitzner, 2008). Because of the urgent nature in managing symptoms, PSM in diabetes developed early, and of all the common chronic diseases has been the most enabled by technology to manage its immediate tasks such as glucose monitoring, insulin delivery, and food and exercise management. For this chronic disease, PSM is not a choice but a necessity in achieving glycemic control.

Diabetes-specific numeracy (the ability to use and understand numbers in daily life) remains problematic because SM requires individuals to accurately calculate and adjust insulin doses, count carbohydrates, calculate portion sizes from food labels, and interpret glucose meter readings. However, a diabetes-specific numeracy test measuring such skills does exist. Tested in a group, more than half the participants had difficulty with addition, subtraction, integer multiplication, and recognition of numerical hierarchy, even though many had adequate health literacy (White, Osborn, Gebretsadik, Kripalani, & Rothman, 2011). While further testing of the instrument is necessary, these findings draw attention to the need to assess numeracy in diabetes SM, especially in this context where safety requires more rigorous skills.

Studies of persons with diabetes raise some of the same identity issues as were raised by persons with arthritis. To support PSM for this chronic illness, it is essential for providers and patients to think beyond adherence to treatment and recognize SM activities as an identity project. Minet, Lonvig, Henriksen, and Wagner's (2011) study of how patients do this includes narratives about handling diabetes in everyday life, and through peer activity, construction of a norm for appropriate management of diabetes, as well as a sense of self that is capable of meeting SM challenges. Thus, PSM requires that different life demands from different areas of life be integrated into a whole (Minet et al., 2011).

Insulin pens reduce risk of over- and under-dosing and are now available with a memory. While insulin pumps mimic the pattern of insulin release from the pancreas, their use requires patients to make frequent decisions based on insulin pharmacodynamics and carbohydrate counting. New technology aims to improve accuracy of blood glucose self-monitoring. But the optimal replacement therapy for diabetes is a closed-loop system (the artificial pancreas) integrating three elements: continuous or repeated measurement of glucose, a computer that controls insulin delivery, and an insulin infusion pump to maintain a normal glycemic range.

Because it addresses the problem of nocturnal hypoglycemia, overnight closed-loop delivery is particularly important. Theoretically, the artificial pancreas will free patients from SM and optimally manage both short- and long-term complications of diabetes. Data transmission to health care staff computers through radio services and secured web sites allows easy telemonitoring and teleconsultations (Penfornis, Personeni, & Borot, 2011).

Beyond the technology, understanding the dilemmas patients face in living with hypoglycemia is essential to working through SM. A qualitative study found patients believed that health care providers were not concerned about the amount of responsibility involved in avoiding and managing hypoglycemia and focused instead on maintenance of blood sugar levels. Patients understood that an episode of hypoglycemia made them completely dependent on others and unable to care for themselves, and it could also trigger seizures and behavioral changes. These possibilities affected their self-image. Some were hesitant to talk about these issues with their health care providers, fearing they had done something wrong. Individuals indicated they felt only fear and anxiety when faced with the threat of hypoglycemia and were unable to resolve how to deal with it (Wu, Juang, & Yeh, 2011). A competent PSM program should have resolved these issues.

Diabetes is heavily managed in primary care, where up to two-thirds of patients have HbA1c greater than 7%. Perhaps because of the time-consuming nature of insulin therapy for type 2 diabetes, this treatment intensification commonly occurs when patients reach HbA1c levels far in excess of recommended treatment targets. This means that many patients with type 2 diabetes may spend the majority of the duration of their disease with suboptimal glycemic control. Although insulin injection and titration are time intensive for both patient and provider, patient self-titration has been shown in controlled trials to be at least as effective and safe as physician-directed titration and likely more cost effective. But this SM requires patients to be skilled in performing blood glucose monitoring dose calculation and insulin injection (Brunton et al., 2011).

As noted in these accounts, the existing primary care structure is overstretched and under-resourced and so commonly fails to provide optimal care for patients with chronic illness. There is an urgent need to understand how much of this care can be provided by patients in a cost-effective manner (Brunton et al., 2011). Indeed, improvement in the quality of care requires this answer.

SUMMARY

For all these common chronic diseases, PSM is not an option for exacerbations that are serious, even though patients frequently do not know how to detect them, and symptoms like pain must be dealt with. Patient beliefs about chronic disease and its treatment are always important as they may facilitate or block treatment and PSM. For all the diseases outlined here, patient capability to SM has been found effective, sometimes at modest levels. Recently, in some instances (e.g., cancer), treatment administration has migrated to patients, creating a whole new set of SM expectations. However, SM of comorbidities that sometimes accompany these diseases cannot be overlooked.

STUDY QUESTIONS AND ANSWERS

1. It is crucial to remember that diagnostic categories are abstractions we have created, not entities we have discovered in nature (Parens & Johnston, 2009). Why is this insight ethically important?

    Answer: It provides correction of at least two ethically problematic practices/ways of thinking: (a) patients don't have to be stuffed into culturally determined diagnostic categories to receive our attention, and (b) we may forget that expression of elements of a diagnostic category vary (sometimes greatly) across patients, requiring different SM plans/practices.

2. Critics say patients have always either had to practice SM of chronic disease or chose to do this. So, from an ethical/policy point of view, what's new about the current PSM movement?

    Answer: A couple of things are new. First, different means can emphasize different values. Assuming the old SM was about following the doctor's orders, the new SM recognizes important different values such as patient agency and choice of lifestyle and the sometimes negative quality of medical treatments. These values affirm respect for and engagement of patients. Second, the new SM movement is beginning to recognize both the need for policy changes such as payment for PSM education and support services and to a lesser extent the impact of current social policies on patients' ability to manage their chronic diseases. These policies require patients to understand medical knowledge of their illness and also prove their means to carry out PSM, including sufficient access to health care providers.

3. Medication nonadherence is considered a major problem in SM across a number of chronic diseases and is usually characterized as either voluntary on the part of the patient or due to lack of resources to purchase medications. Other origins include lack of shared understanding between patient and provider of what constitutes medical adherence, or tension between social control and values of autonomy and self-control. A recent study of persons with schizophrenia found that nearly all had stopped their antipsychotic medications for extensive periods of time but resumed taking them when they learned about the effects of relapse (Tranulis, Goff, Henderson, & Freudenreich, 2011). What is the ethical relevance of these various definitions of adherence?

Answer: Traditional definitions of nonadherence "blame the victim." But insights from the Tranulis et al. (2011) study show that achieving appropriate patient compliance is an essential part of learning to self-manage, inviting opportunities for providers to work through lessons learned with the patient. This view respects the patient's developing capacity.

4. Knowledge of cancer diagnosis and treatment among breast and colorectal cancer survivors has been judged deficient; this is critical because clinicians must sometimes rely on patient self-report of their history. Findings from a study showed that 40% of breast cancer survivors and 65% of colorectal cancer survivors were unable to identify their stage of disease, and 7% of breast cancer survivors and 21% of colorectal cancer survivors in whom regional nodes were examined did not know whether they had positive nodes. Accuracy of estrogen and progesterone status among breast cancer survivors was 58% and 39%. About half of each group could not identify drugs they had received, even though these can have lasting side effects (Nissen, Tsai, Blaes, & Swenson, in press). What is the ethical implication of a study that raises such questions?

Answer: This study raises questions about the appropriate standard patients should meet to self-manage their illness. In some respects, the investigation "blames the victim" by assuming that patients in communication with providers should make up for deficiencies in medical record availability, whereas this should be the responsibility of the health care system. A better focused view of PSM entails ongoing management of therapy, symptoms and daily living.

5. As with other areas of health care, there has been a strong emphasis on evidence-based medicine (EBM) to justify (or not) expenditure of resources on PSM, including the necessary preparation and support. There are, however, significant limitations of EBM, some with significant ethical implications. Criticisms of EBM have alleged that it oversimplifies complex problems, that it is only (partially) useful when scientific evidence is incomplete or conflicting, and that evidence from RCTs is almost exclusively based on ideal patients (De Vreese, 2011). What are the ethically significant problems with requiring a definitive evidence base as grounds for providing PSM services?

Answer: There are several: (a) there needs to be a consistent standard for treatment levels of evidence that does not now exist; for example, currently some patients who need surgical procedures will get them with a lower level of evidence than those who need PSM support, and (b) there are other bases on which services should be provided, including policy decisions based on desired levels of solidarity in a society or on philosophy about personal agency or empowerment.

6. Some say that PSM is an old concept that has been reinvented. Persons with diabetes always had to control their blood sugar and those with asthma their ability to breathe. Is there anything new about today's PSM as it is currently understood?

   Answer: I think so. The practice has now become more a matter of patient choice, with one of the most cutting edge topics being how to incorporate patient end goals into measurement instruments. There are more home-based or personal technologies, including information technologies. In addition, a few governments now view PSM as a patient right (part of the patient empowerment movement) or as a way to contain health care costs.

7. If a patient wanted to make a choice between an epistemology (way of thinking) of PSM for asthma or diabetes, what alternatives are there?

   Answer: One approach is to realize that PSM occurs on a continuum. Given the available treatments for the disease and their ability to control physiologic disruptions and symptoms in a particular individual, patients should be able to choose the point on that continuum where they are comfortable practicing PSM and where they feel it will be effective, likely moving up the continuum to more responsibility as they develop skills and judgment—or not. Availability of quick electronic communications with providers or other expert opinions aids this decision.

3

Best Practices in
Patient Self-Management
Preparation and Support

In contrast to traditional patient education, which has limited teaching to information and technical skills, patient self-management (PSM) is problem-focused and action-oriented and emphasizes patient-generated care plans. As described by Iversen, Hammond, and Betteridge (2010), self-management (SM) preparation and support aims to influence health knowledge, attitudes, beliefs, and behaviors in order to promote patients' independence and help them maintain or adjust life roles, thus PSM must address the psychosocial impact of disease. Patients have described PSM as bringing order into their lives, helping them to understand how to mobilize resources and cope with their condition.

What are the elements of capability development to allow responsible PSM functioning, and what are the structures through which this care is delivered? This chapter focuses on intervention strategies that enable PSM, starting with a restructured care system in which disease management is embedded (e.g., Chronic Care Model [CCM]) and proceeding to peer models, clinician/patient interaction, and family support preparation.

CHRONIC CARE MODEL

The CCM represents a redesign of the health care system to improve delivery of ambulatory care, particularly for chronic diseases. It includes support of SM by patients; decision supports for providers; use of patient registries, provider reminders, and feedback; use of clinical information systems; and facilitation for linking provider organizations with community-based resources. Systematic reviews and meta-analyses show that care organized by the CCM is more effective than usual care in management of chronic diseases such as asthma and diabetes. Yet a recent study found that only about half of practices across the United States used these processes in the care of common chronic conditions, and utilization lagged even further in treatment of depression. In fact, there are few data on the comparative effectiveness of the various elements of the CCM across different chronic conditions (Zafar & Mojtabai, 2011). In spite of this lack of evidence, the CCM also forms the basis for the Patient-Centered Medical Home Model (Suter, Hennessey, Florez, & Newton, 2011).

Although the CCM has been disseminated in federally qualified health care centers, its integration into home care has lagged, even though many of our most chronically ill cannot access clinic settings. Indeed, nearly 8 million patients with chronic diseases and other conditions are cared for by home health agencies. Given that the current practice-based health care system in the United States provides no mechanism to assist with ongoing disease monitoring or long-term support, homebound patients and their caregivers continue to bear much of the responsibility for illness management and must be educated for it (Suter et al., 2011).

Fortunately, a recent summary of published evidence suggests that practices redesigned in accord with the CCM generally improve the quality of care and outcomes for patients with various chronic diseases. But most of the studies involved highly motivated practices and focused on patients with a single chronic condition. There is little evidence in these studies to ensure that practice changes are sustained or that the model will spread to those with multi-morbidity or to less motivated practitioners (Coleman, Austin, Brach, & Wagner, 2009).

In addition to the CCM, other organizational configurations have also been found to support PSM and achieve good outcomes. For example, disease management programs at Sutter Health (a California group medical practice) were integrated closely with diabetes SM education services. Assessment of patient knowledge occurred at the time of enrollment in the diabetes management program, with prompt referrals to the diabetes educator if needed. The disease management staff then reinforced skills learned in the education course. Sutter Health illustrates that a clinical information system (i.e., diabetes registry) is essential to such a program. The provider reveals that collaboration between disease management and diabetes education services can be used for subpopulations, for instance, women with high risk pregnancies including gestational diabetes, with postpartum follow up to determine if the patient has type 2 diabetes. At Sutter Health, RNs and clinical pharmacists were available 24 hours a day, 7 days a week to support the disease management program and provide PSM support for healthier moms and babies (Fitzner et al., 2008).

In another example of health care restructuring, an effort to reduce 30-day re-hospitalization rates (currently at 20% to 25% for those over age 65), Care Transitions Intervention (CTI) provided transition coaches for high risk patients. CTI focused on empowering these patients to better manage their illnesses through home visits and telephone calls, helping patients to understand signs and symptoms of any worsening of their condition and preparing them to self-manage and communicate effectively with their providers. A randomized controlled trial of CTI showed a reduction of 30-day hospital readmission rates by 30% compared with a control group (Voss et al., 2011). But although useful, such an intervention is very time limited and assumes that PSM support will continue with the patient's community-based providers—not a valid assumption.

As a final example of restructured care, let us consider a suggestion for transformative innovation in hypertension management. Less than half of hypertensive patients in America have their blood pressure treated to guideline-recommended target goals. A series of steps necessary to improve this statistic includes the following: improving patient engagement and communication with providers, increasing the use of nonphysician providers, better provider performance monitoring and feedback systems, and better aligned health care reimbursement models. This transformative model is presented in Table 3.1 and includes enhanced PSM with regular downloading of data to and communication with the provider. Blood pressure self-monitoring stations are currently located throughout communities but should be expanded to churches, grocery stores, salons, and barber shops. The current system of periodic physician office visits offers an incentive to see the patient but not to control his or her blood pressure, and therefore may create lags in management of the condition (Roark, Shah, Udayakumar, & Peterson, 2011).

TABLE 3.1
Expanding Hypertension Management

Model	Intervention	Outcome
Self-management	Home and remote blood pressure monitoring Self-education Personalized goal setting	Improved blood pressure control Improved weight loss Increased monitoring of blood pressure
Nonphysician clinical providers	Lifestyle and diet modification Medication titration Increased guideline adherence Extension of provider services	Diet and lifestyle improvements Improved weight loss Improved blood pressure control Increased access to primary care services More rapid blood pressure goal attainment
Telemedicine/ web-based care	Remote monitoring of blood pressure Telephone-based behavioral intervention Disease management hotlines Web-based risk assessment Web-based lifestyle and behavioral interventions	Increased monitoring of blood pressure More cost-effective educational intervention programs Improved risk assessment Increased access to primary care services Increased interactions with health care team
Nonclinic-based care	Blood pressure kiosks in grocery stores, barber shops, churches, and other public places Community health workers	Increased ability to check and monitor blood pressure Improved patient engagement Increased awareness Care provided closer to patient's home
Provider monitoring and feedback	Clinical outcomes data tracked for providers, hospitals, and health systems Comparative analyses completed for providers Information released publicly	Improved clinical outcomes Physician benchmarking by providers, payers, and patients Quality improvement by physicians

Source: Adapted from Roark, Udayakumar, & Peterson (2011), *American Heart Journal*, *162*, pp. 405–411. Copyright © American Heart Association. Used with permission of Mosby, Inc., via Copyright Clearance Center.

In summary, the examples presented so far demonstrate how lack of PSM is in part a system problem.

STRUCTURED PROGRAMS INCLUDING PEER MODELS

Other approaches to implement PSM preparation and support can be provided by health professionals or by peers, in programs of various levels of structure.

An excellent example of a structured program is reported by Hamnes, Hauge, Kjeken, and Hagen (2011) and colleagues at Lillehammer Hospital for Rheumatic Diseases in Norway. A 1-week program led by a multidisciplinary team used an empowering approach and included themes such as diseases and treatment, pain and stress management, exercise and nutrition, assessment of one's own resources and limitations, values and choices, and personal goals. The program also provided exercises to learn how to manage fatigue. The entire program focused on meeting patient expectations, which included helping them assume more responsibility for and acceptance of their disease, helping employed patients continue in their jobs, and helping all patients to communicate effectively about their situation. Several persons in this program expressed the hope that it would help them break the daily circle of perceived pain, fatigue and lack of coping (Hamnes et al., 2011).

Peer support is an approach to care that provides emotional, appraisal, and informational assistance via a created social network member who possesses experiential knowledge and social characteristics similar to the target population. The support, which may arrive as peer coaching or mentoring, involves individuals who usually have the same condition as their assigned patient and who work with the peer on a less structured basis than traditional health care professionals while providing emotional support and serving as a role model. These programs are predominantly group-based or implemented by telephone or Internet. The most favorable findings from these interventions are for greater self-efficacy, fewer depressive symptoms, and higher quality of life (for diabetes-specific interventions) when compared with usual-care control groups. Although peer-led interventions require training and logistical support, they may serve a vital role in low-resource settings where access to health professionals is scarce (Tang, Guadalupe, Cherrington, & Rana, 2011).

Key functions of peer support for diabetes management may be found in Table 3.2 (Fisher Earp, Maman, & Zolotor, 2010).

TABLE 3.2
Key Functions of Peer Support for Diabetes Management

Behavioral Objectives	Specific Operational Approaches to Behavioral Objectives	Outcome/Measurement
Key function: assistance in managing and living with diabetes in daily life		
Assist problem solving to support regimen adherence in daily life	• Use problem-solving intervention techniques • Share stories of challenges and success • Assist in changing routines or other adjustments to facilitate adherence	• Audits of topics covered • Participant reports of types of interactions addressing problem solving • Participant reports of management tasks addressed
Engage in healthy eating, physical activity together	• Share regular modest physical activity (e.g., walking, swimming, tennis, others) • Share in healthy eating behaviors (e.g., shop for food, prepare meals, and/or eat meals together)	• Participant reports of shared activities • Physical activity • Healthy eating • Others
Key function: social and emotional support		
Maintain frequent contact	• Face-to-face contact • Telephone contact • Electronic contact (web, email, text message)	• Contact records or reports
Encourage, enhance motivation	• Point out progress • Reassure of long-term nature of diabetes management • Reassure that medical care and medications can help • Reassure that one is "doing one's best"	• Audits of topics covered • Participant reports of support received/provided using standard measures

TABLE 3.2
Key Functions of Peer Support for Diabetes Management *(continued)*

Behavioral Objectives	Specific Operational Approaches to Behavioral Objectives	Outcome/Measurement
Provide support in dealing with day-to-day stressors	• Use problem-solving intervention techniques • Share stories of challenges and successes • Be available to listen and discuss problems	• Audits of topics covered • Participant reports of types of interactions addressing problem solving
Tailoring of support to regional and cultural practices and settings	• Consideration of national, regional, and cultural differences in social support, preferences for types and styles of social support • Providing support that is tuned to individual, social, and cultural features	• Interviews with program staff and peers to characterize key features of support within their settings and cultures • Participant ratings of their satisfaction with peer support provided and the extent to which support is easily accepted
Advocate for and represent those with diabetes	• Serve on advisory committees • Encourage individuals and groups to assert their needs with health providers, community organizations	• Program documentation of committee and advisory roles Advocacy activities
Ethical considerations	• Consideration of individual rights and privacy and limits on roles of peer support within the contexts of difference countries, cultures, and settings	• Documentation of ethical issues emergent through individual projects • Participant ratings of being treated with consideration for their rights, privacy, etc.

(continued)

TABLE 3.2
Key Functions of Peer Support for Diabetes Management *(continued)*

Behavioral Objectives	Specific Operational Approaches to Behavioral Objectives	Outcome/Measurement
Key function: linkage to clinical care		
Develop and maintain linkages with care providers	• Organize peer support within primary care or other principal source of clinical care • Maintain active linkages with providers of primary and clinical care such as by referral, meetings to discuss key issues, training, etc.	• Characterization of linkages with primary care and systems of care • Audits of key interactions (e.g., number referrals to peer support, training of peer supporters) between support and care providers • Participant ratings of extent to which peer support is connected to sources of care
Encourage regular clinical care, partnership with clinical providers	• Remind each other of times for regular physician visits • Encourage physician visits when circumstances or symptoms warrant • Coordination with clinical practices and guidelines within country and setting	• Audits of topics covered • Participant reports of regular, out-patient clinical care

Source: Adapted from Fisher, Earp, Maman, & Zolotor (2010), *Family Practice*, *27*(Suppl 1), pp. 6–16. Copyright © Oxford University Press. Used with permission via Copyright Clearance Center.

The best studied peer-led programs include the Asthma and Chronic Disease Self-Management Programs developed by Lorig and colleagues, which use behavioral goal setting, problem solving, and social support as strategies for coping with negative feelings and to build self-efficacy. Building on this model, the National Health Service in the United Kingdom launched the Expert Patient Programme in 2001. A number of evaluations showed significant improvement in participants' chronic disease management self-efficacy; however, there is still need for rigorous research to document other outcomes. Qualitative evaluations revealed that peer support and learning were two perceived strengths of these programs (Wilson, 2008).

Empowerment-based programs use a similar approach, with clinical content provided by health professional facilitators in response to questions and issues raised by group members. A caveat is that such programs may be specific to cultural groups. Unfortunately, many peer-based programs do not clearly identify the behavioral strategies used by minority peers, and little is known about a successful training program for diverse groups, including about their supervision or about the ways in which the mentoring peer is also helped (Funnell, 2010).

Still, one example of the particular strength of peers is in dealing with patient resistance to initiation or intensification of insulin therapy. Many patients are afraid of giving themselves an injection due to potential hypoglycemia; in addition, insulin may represent treatment failure, social stigma, and advancing illness. Findings indicate that patients may benefit from discussing such concerns with another person who has successfully coped with insulin management (Heisler, 2010).

It is important to note that some patients may not want peer mentoring or support, particularly group support. They may have concerns about privacy and confidentiality, and/or they may not believe they have the social skills or self-confidence to participate. The less motivated may just not want to attend. On the other hand, people obtain both normative guidance and model behaviors through comparisons with similar others, commonly assessing the appropriateness of their own attitudes, beliefs, and behaviors against those modeled in the group. Individuals will often shift to match others in the group, which can include either risky or preventive behaviors, attitudes, and beliefs. On a positive note, similar social characteristics boost the utility of the experience-based support that peer members provide. These individuals provide emotional support, information, advice, feedback, and coping encouragement (Thoits, 2011). An example is seen in diabetes PSM, in which peer support interventions were found to improve glycemic control, healthy eating, patient activation, self-efficacy, and communication with physicians (Lynch & Egede, 2011).

In the above examples, peer education/support is embedded in structured programs. The current literature suggests there is much not yet studied about community-based social networks outside formal health care settings that may either support or undermine PSM. Still, some studies have indicated that social networks, currently considered only as part of the social context in programs that focus on individuals, play a central role in both PSM success and the creation of inequalities. They provide (or don't provide) crucial information and narratives that define normalcy or deviance, notions of individual responsibility, and referrals (Vassilev, 2011).

In fact, social networks that include members with or without crucial information (in this case, about the option of kidney transplant) make a difference in understanding why Black dialysis patients in the United States are less likely than Whites to be evaluated and listed for a kidney transplant. Augmenting the social networks of disadvantaged patients with more knowledgeable individuals is a largely unused intervention strategy (Browne, 2011). Social media offer such an opportunity, but one that is frequently missed. As an example, only a few women with urinary incontinence seek the attention of health professionals, as the condition is largely self-managed. But a study of Facebook, Twitter and YouTube on this topic found little that was informative, with only a small fraction of information provided by incontinence professionals or organizations heavily oriented to protective pads or undergarments and ignoring other treatments (Sajadi & Goldman, 2011).

As a final patient group to note, people with intellectual disabilities are four times more likely than the general population to have a chronic disease and so should be served by SM programs. Such a program has been developed by redesigning each session of the generic Expert Patients Programme and incorporating information on the long-term conditions commonly affecting this user group (such as epilepsy). The tutor's manual, aimed specifically at facilitating groups made up of people with intellectual disabilities, and DVDs were produced using actors with intellectual disabilities. A prerequisite for attending the program was having the social skills that allowed functioning within a group. In subsequent program improvements, the language was simplified and the course was run 2 weeks longer. This course has been piloted (Wilson & Goodman, 2011) and represents a good faith effort to reach the diverse group of people who need to learn SM. Their capabilities can be developed.

PROVIDER-PATIENT INTERACTION

PSM preparation and support can be supplied as part of the provider-patient interaction and/or by structured self-managed interventions that include protocols with handbooks. In either case, in comparison with patient education, these interventions are problem-focused and action-oriented, and they emphasize patient-generated care plans. For example, patients with arthritis have been found to view such interventions as a way to bring order into their lives, help them mobilize resources, cope with change in self-identity (further explored in Chapter 4), and plan, pace, and prioritize life goals. Psychobehavioral SM interventions have been documented to lead to short term (6–9 month) benefits, but are often not evaluated for longer-term benefits and furthermore are rarely sustained. In addition, there is little research on who benefits most from SM interventions (Iversen et al., 2010).

Other studies suggest the importance of a relationship with a health provider for emotional support as the patient constructs his or her own individual SM program. Furler et al.'s (2008) study showed individuals learning to self-manage diabetes and to deal with the emotional highs and lows of their chronic condition while understanding that neglect of SM would result in deteriorating health. The patients felt a sense of resentment that enjoyable aspects of life had been unjustly removed by this disease, and as a result of the diagnosis distrusted their bodies. A feeling of coping with loss was palpable among the patients of this study, who looked to health professionals and SM strategies to exert control over their condition. These findings underscore that living with self-managed diabetes is as much a social and emotional task as a technical task (Furler et al., 2008).

Much has been made of another interaction approach to engage patients in PSM, motivational interviewing (MI). MI can be characterized as a style or spirit of being with patients rather than a mere application of techniques. An example is seen in patients with chronic kidney disease who, as the disease progresses, experience an increase in PSM demands frequently accompanied by wavering of motivation. Practitioners attend to the balance of patient statements that seem to support or thwart behavior change in order to gauge patient motivation and adjust their own use of MI techniques, which include rolling with resistance, expressing empathy, developing discrepancy between the patient's current behavior and important values or goals, and supporting the patients' self-efficacy to believe they can change their behavior. In MI, practitioners reflect aloud the discrepancy between the way the patient wants to be and the pathways taken, explore with patients how behavior change might help them achieve their self-perceptions and goals, and pay particular attention to their patients' past successful change efforts. Ethically, MI is meant to express respect for patients and support of their autonomy and capacity to make decisions and initiate change. A summary of MI studies showed it to exert small but clinically significant effects (Martino, 2011).

In summary, the provider-patient relationship is essential to PSM of chronic disease but frequently problematic because it is embedded in the incentives of the current health care system. Fortunately, we are blessed with an exceptional set of analyses that point very clearly to the immense opportunities for meaningful reform in order to properly care for patients with chronic disease. These analyses also carry the message that unless providers are able to leap over these disincentives and unuseful attitudes, management of patients with chronic disease, including the inevitable PSM, will remain problematic.

Thorne's (2006) analysis is especially prescient.

"... Persons with chronic illness are not high-priority patients, there is little that can be offered that will make a difference in their lives ... unchecked, they will use up more than their fair share of health resources.

... Although persons with chronic illness report being confronted on a daily basis with the limits of science for answering the immediate questions of how to live life with their particular condition, the healthcare professional sector still functions, for the most part, as if scientific expertise is its singular prerogative and the ultimate source of all meaningful and pertinent knowledge...

... The work of learning a chronic illness is much less about accessing and interpreting scientific information than it is about analyzing the relevance of that information to a unique set of manifestations and responses ... through body listening and experimentation, not standardized protocols.

Chronically ill persons can become trapped in double binds when they are simultaneously trying to seek appropriate support while normalizing their conditions ... Most encounter disrespectful, discrediting and distressing healthcare communications at some point in their illness careers.

Newly diagnosed chronically ill patients typically ... assume that modern medicine will cure their problems. When communication tensions go unresolved, a struggle for control often ensues with regard to who has ultimate authority in managing the illness ... physician rendering orders and the patient failing to comply ... "

Others have focused on the shared decision making (SDM) that is essential in chronic care and is now becoming policy in many jurisdictions. A study of such interactions found that because mutual and independent patient reflection rarely took place in traditional settings, patients and professionals seldom accomplished joint insight into how a particular illness therapy could integrate life-oriented and disease-oriented perspectives. Most treatment activities were disease-oriented and centered on patient symptoms and the results of tests and treatment, rather than taking a life-oriented stance and focusing on a particular patient's reactions to diabetes in daily life with other people. Interestingly, these difficulties actually seemed to disempower patients and professionals; in contrast, shared knowledge can empower and strengthen the relationship (Zoffmann, Harder, & Kirkevold, 2008).

Even the notion of error can be ambiguous in chronic disease management. For example, in diabetes care, there is no single correct treatment; instead notions of optimal treatments unfold over time after iterative attempts to improve. In this context, not trying things could be interpreted as more mistaken than unanticipated adverse consequences, which in other circumstances might be labeled as errors. The failure to continue to try and improve treatment and life adjustment might reflect an error of aspiration for the patient. But the economy of clinic visits can also create errors of investment, placing constraints on provider capacity to engage in these processes of discovery and iterative patient support for PSM. The active role of patients in chronic care creates a strong framework for attributing treatment shortcomings to the patients and away from providers, even though some findings may be due to progression of the disease. As a related issue, providers are held responsible for reaching explicit targets that may conflict directly with the individualization necessary to treat these patients (Lutfey & Freese, 2007).

The new standard of SDM is clearly a revolution in the making. Widely accepted as a new standard and developed initially for acute care decision making, questions about how the concept can work for chronic disease remain. How should preferences of patient and provider be weighed? Several studies show how difficult this is to accomplish. Shortus, Kemp, McKenzie, and Harris (in press) found providers sought to actively manage the patient's involvement in decision making according to what they hoped to achieve, believing beneficence in treating a patient's diabetes to target was more important than bending these targets to support the patient's autonomy. Sometimes staff members, such as diabetes educators, get caught in the middle of this tussle. Some providers deliberately sought to limit patient involvement in care planning to prevent too much deviation from best practice guidelines (Shortus et al., in press).

Other studies show physician annoyance if patients insisted on their preferences and doubted the doctor's recommendation, or searched the Internet for other patients' experiences (Hamann et al., in press). In a study of provision of asthma care, SDM was used as a tool to support the nurse's agenda rather than as a true provider-patient partnership, giving the patient only the illusion of power (Upton et al., 2011).

Talk about a set of disincentives and mismatches! A crucial question to ask is, can they be put right? As shown by evidence, absolutely; and addressing them is important in achieving PSM. At a deeper level of ethical analysis, a cluster of illustrations from Norwegian authors suggests that modern medical practice precludes attending to patients' existential concerns and the accompanying suffering. Although their cases feature doctors and hospitalized patients, it is highly likely that the same mode of practice is used in ambulatory chronic disease management. These doctors actively directed the focus away from patients' personal concerns of being recently widowed or worrying about surgery, with the rejection of these concerns likely producing moral harm. The physicians were courteous but attended only to medical knowledge, such as declaring a patient's health on the basis of a test result, and overlooking the patient's own account of his life. Such a practice mode risks being less effective (Agledahl Gulbrandsen, Forde, & Wifstad, 2011), leaving patients confused as to whether they are worthy of the kind of capability development that could occur by addressing these existential concerns.

FAMILY AND COMMUNITY SUPPORT

Patients often grapple with the intricate details of revised SM goals and instructions, medication changes, and medical testing. Programs to prepare family members to support PSM include those that: (a) guide family members in setting goals for supporting patient SM behaviors, (b) train family in supportive communication such as use of autonomy supportive statements or prompting patient coping techniques, and (c) give families tools to assist in monitoring clinical symptoms and medications. Currently, little evidence is available on the impact of these programs (Rosland & Piette, 2010).

A confluence of issues in management of chronic disease makes families/groups/cultures central to PSM. First, medicine's focus on the individual body does not consider the social context in which the many daily decisions/actions of PSM take place, and success of medical treatments, largely drugs, has been limited. Because multiple, often opposing, lifestyles cannot be disconfirmed by medical science, groups and individuals make choices about what health is and how to achieve it, which in turn, may be disapproved by some individual medical practitioners. Thus within the context of families and cultural groups, beliefs and choices are made on the basis of available knowledge and options within a market-based health care system. Medicine becomes only one voice among many and its current style of practice and episteme disconnected from real life (Wasserman & Hinote, 2011), leading us to the need for a nursing model based on longitudinal development of patient/family/community capabilities.

Multigenerational legacies of diabetes include patients connecting their family members' experiences with SM and onset of complications with their own subsequent decisions about SM influenced by perceptions of controllability and consequences of the disease and its treatment with insulin. Exploring these perceptions and related emotions of fear or sadness during educational sessions is important, as legacies of diabetes may include myths or stories passed through families that may or may not be accurate. A recent study found emotional representations were prominent among patients in this situation (Scollan-Koliopoulos, Walker, & Rapp, 2011).

Given the tremendously increasing rates of diabetes, especially in ethnic minority populations, community-based PSM programs are essential in nonhealth settings such as churches and community centers and often include community health workers (CHWs) on the team. CHWs have a close understanding of the community served; and they can ensure cultural competence in the service delivered and build community capabilities through education, informed counseling, and advocacy (Fitzner, Dietz, & Moy, 2011).

AN ALTERNATIVE NURSING MODEL

Where nursing specialist roles have developed, as in management of diabetes or, to a lesser extent, asthma, evidence indicates these practitioners do well in preparing and supporting PSM in chronic diseases and in broader roles (e.g., nurse practitioners) as the primary care provider for these patients. For example, in the United Kingdom, most patients with airway diseases are now managed in primary care by nurses working with general practitioners, a major transformation. Precipitated by a change in the payment system, the number of nurses practicing in expanded roles has grown rapidly; at the same time, it is essential to ensure that they are adequately trained and certified (Upton et al., 2007).

These and other developments raise a more basic suggestion. As currently practiced, the medical model and incentive systems to support it do not sustain the level of patient agency and attention to social/life aspects of chronic disease necessary to efficiently manage the chronic disease burden. But after decades of work, it is still questionable if the CCM is effective in altering that situation. The dynamic in play seems less than useful—more attempts to get patients to comply with the prescribed regimen and blaming them when they don't (call this compliance essentialism), and continuing evidence that persons with chronic disease don't have the knowledge and access to support that allows success, as well as concern that these deficits contribute to widening health disparities.

An alternative model recognizes the success of specialist roles but constructs a parallel system, driven by the capabilities model outlined in Chapter 1. In this approach, advance practice nurses would automatically manage those with chronic diseases within a defined scope of practice. In some countries like the United Kingdom, certain specialist roles like the diabetes specialist nurse (DSN) have existed for 70 years. A recent survey shows 1,363 DSNs working in the United Kingdom with a recommendation that one should be employed for every 250,000 population set. Preparation for these nurse specialist roles varies by country (James, 2010). Such a health care model would incorporate one more explicitly rooted in nursing, recognizing patient need for meaning and purpose in life and their autonomy, and working with their lived experiences (Porter, O'Halloran, & Morrow, 2011). We can call this the embedded morality of nursing, compelling society toward development of patient capabilities to manage their health issues and lives.

Similarly, oncology specialist nurse roles in the United Kingdom have just evolved but remain poorly evaluated, with great disparities in scope of practice and autonomy and much on-the-job training. Driven by policy changes in cancer services focusing on patient safety during chemotherapy treatment, nurse-led clinics provide routine follow up care (Farrell, Molassiotis, Beaver, & Heaven, 2011).

Likewise, in an effort to reduce the approximately half of preventable hospital admissions in patients with heart failure, specially trained heart failure nurses provide important education, monitoring, and coordination of care among multiple providers in a complex, disjointed health care delivery system in the United States. Especially useful are roles in which the health professional follows the patient to the home in order to detect subtle changes that indicate early decompensation as well as help the patient develop SM skills (Manning, 2011). Such programs appear necessary to support patient safety in heart failure treatment. As an indication of this need, a survey of nurses practicing in 1,406 hospitals in nine countries found that half in every country lacked confidence that patients could care for themselves following discharge (Aiken et al., 2011).

A move to such a nurse-managed model requires us to look at an entirely different set of ethical and practice issues; these are outlined in the chapters that follow. It also requires enforced standards regarding patient ability to self-manage chronic illness. But beyond these essentials, a nurse-managed model requires escape from the patriarchal, medically dominated system under which many nurses have practiced. Such systems force a nurse's clinical judgment into a medical model oriented to disease, patient compliance with the treatment regimen, and physicians as gatekeepers to any PSM education and support services.

As a group, physician practice patterns and philosophy do not embrace PSM; many spend little time on it or do not incorporate PSM education or support competently. At the same time many physicians will not cede education and support to nursing because this would mean loss of income and power. In the medically dominant model, the "good nurse" silences the voice of her own profession and suffers moral conflict because of it. Nurses routinely see incompetent medical practice in the management of chronic disease but do not speak up; they must keep up the façade that physicians are essential to this work when in truth they are not. It is easy to be led down the path of fully internalizing these myths. So what is a new direction?

The way out is for nursing to take leadership in partnership with patients, to define goals of PSM (beyond compliance with the medical regimen as an end goal) and to straighten out the muddled constructs inherent in this practice. Nursing models of practice are much more in tune with patient perception and experience, focusing on patient life goals into which disease/symptom management is incorporated, not vice versa. Practicing in truly democratic multidisciplinary teams, each practitioner and patient contributing skills and challenging the other partner, is the way to go. Recall that education and support is clearly within nursing's legal scope of practice; this creates a positive obligation to allow nursing performance of these duties.

SUMMARY

The primary organizing framework for chronic disease care, the CCM and/or programs with similar elements, includes PSM but focuses largely on coordinating elements of the organization of care. Of structured programs optimizing PSM, those based on peer education have received the most review. Individual providers operating in current health care systems continue to struggle with appropriate partnerships with patients who by necessity must self-manage their multiple chronic illnesses. Invariably, nurse specialist roles are vital when serious attempts at PSM are made, yet standards for these roles are largely underdeveloped, and they operate in a hostile policy environment.

A performance metric for health systems ought to indicate how well people with chronic disease(s) are prepared to care for their condition, solve related problems, and avert complications. Diabetes SM, arguably the best established practice of PSM, is still delivered with great variability in quality and quantity. We do not currently have strong answers for how much PSM support is sufficient, the periodicity of this support, and the comparative effectiveness of various approaches (Schillinger, 2011) described in this chapter.

STUDY QUESTIONS AND ANSWERS

1. Why is a new business model essential for adequate delivery of preparation and support services for PSM of chronic disease?

   Answer: The current U.S. health system has few incentives for this service—almost nonexistent reimbursement, low status among physicians who provide it, and practice guidelines that are widely ignored. A new business model would place advance practice nurses at the center, provide them with reimbursement for reaching patient goals, and allow them to operate independently within their scope of practice.

2. Cognitive impairment is common at some stages of many chronic diseases, affecting memory and executive functions and sometimes predicting mortality. What can be done about it?

   Answer: We should routinely screen for cognitive impairment, being careful to avoid unnecessary labeling. Valid and reliable measures of cognitive impairment are essential for developing successful and safe PSM skills.

3. PSM programs are being reported in China, Finland, Norway, Canada, and many other countries for diseases such as epilepsy, HIV, and back pain (as well as those diseases addressed in this chapter), but study quality assessing their effectiveness has been judged inadequate, and determining the active ingredients of many successful interventions is still unclear (Coster & Norman, 2009). Should these findings be of concern?

   Answer: Yes, they should, because adequate studies are necessary for evidence-based practice guidelines. There are multiple ways to strengthen such studies—establish sensitivity of the instruments to measure SM interventions, describe the level of skills of providers delivering the interventions, and clarify the length of time they must be delivered (Coster & Norman, 2009). Lack of solid effectiveness can be a reason for nonreimbursement of such services. Yet patients have a moral right to this information because chronic disease cannot be successfully managed without their involvement.

4. PSM education and support are frequently provided in groups, inviting social comparisons among participants, especially when people

newly diagnosed with chronic disease feel their lives are out of control. While social comparisons can be helpful (e.g., to gain information from someone with more experience or higher performance), they can also be harmful, inciting increased feelings of lack of control and of hopelessness. How do we make the inevitable social comparisons in groups helpful rather than harmful?

Answer: We can make groups helpful by constructing and managing groups with full awareness that their dynamic has the potential to cause harm. On the other hand, as patients build strong capabilities with high self-efficacy and active coping they become much less vulnerable to potential negative effects of social comparison (Fiske, 2011).

5. Evidence-based medicine, which has been dominant as a criterion for appropriate interventions, has in some studies been found incapable of incorporating patients' values and preferences into clinical decision making. The model is therefore wanting, especially in management of chronic diseases (Miles & Loughlin, 2011). What can replace or at the very least supplement evidence-based practice?

Answer: Miles and Loughlin (2011) suggest personalized models of care informed but not based on evidence, while emphasizing the improbability that information from statistical analyses would routinely be applicable to individual patients. Such a stance supports a model of practice in which interventions that show promise are developed and tried jointly by patient and provider.

6. For some chronic illnesses (e.g., attention-deficit hyperactivity disorder in children), both behavioral and pharmacologic interventions are available, with the latter frequently being favored in current practice. Some ethicists argue that while more time consuming, behavioral interventions not only avoid side effects of medications but more positively teach patients how to control their symptoms over the long haul and thus are more beneficial (Parens & Johnston, 2009). Does this kind of tradeoff occur in a number of chronic diseases?

Answer: Yes. Examples that come to mind include both diabetes and asthma; some patients have considerable difficulty detecting bodily symptoms of deterioration but can be taught this cognizance (glucose awareness training), thus triggering an action plan (an essential part of SM in asthma) to stop a cascade into an emergency that will require more intensive use of drugs.

7. WebEase (Web Epilepsy Awareness, Support and Education) is an online epilepsy SM program to support the development and refinement of SM skills. It incorporates three theoretical perspectives: social cognitive theory, the transtheoretical model of behavior change, and developing MI into modules for medication management, stress management, and sleep management. Participants enter daily information into MyLog, assess their current status, decide whether to change behavior (according to their stage of change), and create a goal and action plan. Content is delivered using MI principles, with patients receiving reflective feedback stating what they said. A discussion board provides a forum for participants to chat with each other. Initial testing for 6 weeks found higher levels of adherence and self-efficacy in this group compared with a wait list control group (Dilorio, Bamps, Walker, & Escoffery, 2011). What critiques can we make of this initial development?

Answer: The program addresses a population who are required to self-manage their chronic condition, but one that is not traditionally included in SM programs. MI can be made available through a mobile phone app, increasing its already good availability through use of the Internet as a delivery mechanism. In its present form the approach uses the best currently known psychosocial theories but misses more patient-oriented outcomes and the exploration of moral dilemmas these patients and their families face.

4

Changing the Patient's Self

Some of the ethical sensitivity needed to properly implement patient self-management (PSM) preparation and support involves recognizing the personal change that accompanies patient learning, particularly when change involves private matters such as an individual's health, lifestyle and socioeconomic status. But in the current health system, indifference to personal evolution has been exacerbated by limited acknowledgment of PSM needs. Patients' complaints often start from the perception that professional or institutional treatment threatens their moral identity as competent, rational, and knowledgeable people, or they discover a harm or potential harm that health professionals didn't disclose, or their requests or warnings are disregarded (Williamson, 2008).

What do these concerns mean specifically in the context of PSM? First, they suggest the opportunity for moral coercion that flows from the power holder's opinions and values. Second, patients may experience increasing disillusionment with professional or institutional beliefs, practices, or standards. Low standards can stay unchanged for a long time, sustained by strong norms as well as by health care professionals' personal choices. Third, the health care community may give only lip service to concepts like patient autonomy, shared decision making, freedom of choice, and safety in self-management (SM) without fully implementing these ideals. Research shows that many patients want more information, choice, respect, and access than they are given (Williamson, 2008).

This chapter addresses patient beliefs and the problems with motivation, concerns with identity and dignity, and moral conflicts patients must resolve to manage a chronic disease. It begins with a discussion of education as initiation into socially constructed norms. The central ethical question that undergirds this chapter's conversation is: How can SM support avoid being seen as an assault on the person and instead focus on building patient capabilities for the long term?

EDUCATION AS INITIATION INTO SOCIALLY CONSTRUCTED NORMS

Education is a platform technology, a basic instrument utilized to help individuals meet societal standards or as a means of changing those standards. Education is also moral practice. It initiates people into worthwhile ways of seeing and experiencing the world and of relating to others. It involves respect for what is worth knowing as well as respect for the learner transformed through learning. Education gives access to ideas and tools through which the learner's distinctive personal development may take place (Pring, 2004).

As such, all education is value laden through interpretation of what should be learned (who ascribes this knowledge and how did it become official) and the assumption that education will change a person for the better; value laden, too, in that education involves an effort to induce beliefs in a way that fully engages the reasoning process of the learner (Collin & Apple, 2010). As a negative effort, indoctrination is a systematic distortion of the teacher's presentation of subject matter, often over a prolonged period of time; this instruction presumably creates a corresponding distortion in learners' understanding. Thus indoctrination is a violation of the autonomy to which persons are entitled (Callan & Arena, 2009). In the tradition of strict patient adherence to a medical regimen, with consequences of abandonment by the health community if the patient doesn't comply, some PSM education/support could be seen as indoctrination.

Although education is present in all cultural institutions to some degree, education of patients has been underdeveloped in traditional health care. It is frequently confused with curricular education in schools and thus marginalized. For example, academic classes teach largely cognitive disciplines with tests for assessing knowledge. Education of patients, on the other hand, should be oriented toward decision making and autonomous actions, and in the spirit of informed consent should protect and display all patient options. In some ways bioethics has been complicit with the view that informed consent, of which one element is comprehension on the part of the patient or research subject, is an unattainable moral standard (Beauchamp, 2010). By implication, other important patient functions such as SM also are unattainable. Yet, learning and teaching theory suggest otherwise. Acknowledging that changes in beliefs, motivation, knowledge of the disease, and skill in its treatment regimen impact patient identity is crucial to understanding the journey self-managers need to travel.

It is important to note that in today's world of instantaneous communication and education, ability to develop human agency is essential. Efficient, self-regulating individuals are able to gain knowledge, skills and self-efficacy (SE); deficiencies in these traits can limit self-development (Bandura, 2006). Indeed, such self-direction is a kind of meta-capability—a means for developing the capabilities outlined in Chapter 1 and necessary for sustained PSM.

BELIEFS

The predominant research focus assumes that patient beliefs are highly predictive of compliance with a prescribed medical regimen, with discrepancies between lay (patient) and professional beliefs predictive of noncompliance. Two theoretical models are heavily used to understand patient beliefs. The most prominent is Leventhal, Yael, and Shafers's (2007) common sense model (self-regulatory theory) with five components of beliefs: (1) identity of the illness (symptoms, labels), (2) time-line (acute or chronic), (3) causes (genes, exposure to viruses, etc.), (4) control (can it be prevented, cured, or controlled), and (5) consequences (pain, dysfunction, economic and social losses). Kaptein and Broadbent (2007) summarize instruments used to measure these components.

The health belief model, which is seldom used to understand perceptions of illness, taps patient perceptions of susceptibility to a health condition, severity should they get the disease, and the benefits and barriers to action frequently precipitated by cues. Regardless of which model is applied, essential to all health actions is the belief of SE, or the confidence that one can accomplish what needs to be done (Bandura, 2007).

Lay knowledge goes beyond empirical medical knowledge, incorporating personal experiences and cultural knowledge to support the wider framework of interpretation needed to make coherent sense of the illness (Williams & Popay, 2006). These two forms of knowledge—lay and medical—will always be in tension. Reconciling them by changing the patient's beliefs to conform to medical knowledge frequently leads to better patient compliance with a prescribed regimen. An example of lay knowledge is the belief that because symptoms are temporary, an illness such as asthma or depression is not chronic and does not require ongoing medication. As another example, researchers have studied the cultural belief among African Americans that hypertension is caused by stress. Yet through patient education, a medical belief model of hypertension controlled by factors such as diet, age, and weight was associated with lower systolic blood pressure (Hekler et al., 2008).

In order to guide belief systems, it has been suggested that health professionals routinely assess the patient's perception of illness. As a case in point, Petrie, Cameron, Ellis, Buick, and Weinman (2002) have shown that after myocardial infarction, an in-hospital intervention to change lay beliefs to conform to the medical model yielded (in comparison with a control group) the patient feeling better prepared to leave the hospital as well as a faster return to work and fewer angina symptoms. The intervention format was basically individualized teaching customized according to the patient's responses to the Illness Perception Questionnaire, exploring patient beliefs about the illness, developing an action plan for minimizing future risk, increasing beliefs of SE, helping the patient distinguish symptoms of normal healing from those that constitute warning signs, and resolving patient concerns about medications.

Another example is seen in patient beliefs about chronic pain. Such beliefs are predictive of outcome and may be modified by educational interventions that increase patient knowledge of pain management strategies, correct misconceptions, and increase patient feelings of control (Vallerand, Templin, Hasenau, & Riley-Doucet, 2007). Or consider people with asthma who frequently believe that if symptoms are absent, they no longer have the disorder (no symptoms, no asthma disease belief) and that medications work better if not used all the time. Research has found that these beliefs are related to poorer response to symptoms. In a small study of children, those with more sophisticated asthma beliefs and management had beneficial changes over 18 months in asthma-related biological profiles—decreased eosinophil counts, improved lung function, and increased daily cortisol output (Walker & Chen, 2010).

Forms of respectful intervention to change beliefs include titration of medication paced by the patient, or joint construction with the provider of a therapeutic narrative to describe their chronic illness experience in order to facilitate a long-term treatment alliance. What none of these studies acknowledge, however, is that illness narratives and beliefs carry moral considerations connecting family background and biographical events, notions of shame and blame, and the need to reconstruct coherence in patients' life histories. Careful analysis of beliefs about causes of illness clarifies what is at stake for the patient. The autoimmunity theory of systemic lupus erythematosus, for example, was often seen as a self-destructive process, somewhat akin to suicide. In other words, in correcting patient belief systems the appropriation of biomedical theories is not straightforward (Taieb et al., 2010).

Traditional models of patient decision making assume rational choice. Yet providers frequently meet patient irrationalities that contravene their long-term goals. These include being influenced by what is most readily available in memory, inaccurate projections of future states, and preferring the path already taken in favor of other paths that might clearly produce better results but require change of habit or health resources. Some theorists suggest that in cases where there is only one clear medically favorable choice, clinicians use beneficent persuasion to influence patient decision making. But what if the best decision for a specific patient is less certain? Clinicians could make the patient aware of his or her decisional biases so as to enhance autonomous choice, or perhaps negotiate a trial of the treatment. Less appropriate might be persuasive techniques such as showing videos in the waiting room of children who have suffered from not being vaccinated (to offset parents' concerns about risks of vaccination), or encouraging patients to anticipate regret if they continue to smoke and then develop lung cancer (Swindell, McGuire, & Halpern, 2010). Certainly, irrationalities should be addressed with patients; less clear are the limits that should be placed on provider persuasive techniques.

Beliefs stemming from providers and the institutions in which care is given form a prevailing logic. Each belief has a moral component and a factual component, the falsity of which can distort moral judgment. The greater the moral risks of believing something, the higher the evidentiary burden (Buchanan, 2007). Consider these prevailing logics about PSM and then identify their ethical and factual errors:

- People of low education don't want to and/or cannot learn PSM.
- PSM is optional with chronic diseases.
- Physicians should make decisions about who is able and ready to self-manage.
- Providers and health care institutions don't have an obligation to make PSM preparation and support available in the amount necessary for successful implementation.
- Research must indicate that PSM is superior to provider-based care.
- PSM is always harmless to patient safety and identity.
- Capability development over the long haul is unimportant and too expensive.

One could surmise that a significant reason PSM has not been recognized and developed is because the false beliefs outlined above have been sustained due to an exaggerated sense of physician expertise. The privileges that accompany medical elitism keep others from challenging their authority. For each of these false beliefs, however, there is empirical evidence to the contrary; not only that, but patients (and nurses whose practice involves providing PSM support) are a font of illuminating experiential knowledge that should be acknowledged. In contrast, it is easy to see how false beliefs of this sort can be morally damaging to patients and providers alike.

What happens to patients who refuse to convert to biomedical beliefs? If they are reluctant to comply with medical regimens, they will be under pressure to do so, likely causing psychological distress and potential alienation from their health care providers who, in turn, are under pressure to produce recognized treatment outcomes. In these situations, additional approaches to motivate behavioral change must be considered.

MOTIVATION

Two current approaches to motivation are congruent with the notion of capacity building in patients learning to self-manage their chronic disease. Social-cognitive theory posits that effective PSM requires development of self-regulatory skills on how to influence one's own motivation and behavior. Central and pervasive to PSM is a belief in personal efficacy. In social-cognitive theory, stress arises from perceived inefficacy to exercise control over aversive threats. PSM requires not only skills but a resilient sense of efficacy, developed through goal-setting, problem-solving, and self-diagnostic effort yielding success, and through watching others do the same (Bandura, 2006).

No matter what other factors may serve as motivators, they are rooted in the core belief that one has the power to effect changes by one's actions (SE). SE helps people persevere in the face of adversities, decreases vulnerability to stress and depression, and influences individuals' willingness to select more challenging goals. Most importantly, SE helps people learn to manage their capacities (thoughts, engagement with learning) in order to believe in themselves as autonomous, self-regulated learners. Frequently, patients get "stuck" in their journey to SM, unable to figure out why what they are doing is not working and what to do about it (Parajes, 2008). SE helps the patient break that cycle.

Motivational interviewing (MI), first introduced in Chapter 3, is becoming the most prominent approach to stimulating patient motivation. Developed with addictive conditions such as alcohol and drug abuse, MI is now being applied to a wide range of health behaviors including diet, exercise, and safe sex. A meta-analysis of 119 studies showed small effect sizes when judged against weak (e.g., giving a pamphlet or wait-list) comparison groups, with smaller effect sizes judged against specific treatments (Lundahl, Kunz, Brownell, Tollefson, & Burke, 2010). MI involves providers expressing empathy, developing discrepancy so that clients can argue against themselves about why they should change, rolling with resistance so that reluctance to change is seen as normal, and supporting clients' SE in their ability to change. MI is presented as having a humanistic philosophy and being collaborative in nature, defined by strong rapport between professional and client (Lundahl et al., 2010).

MI is an alternative to a directive style on the part of the provider, which is believed to generate resistance or passivity in the patient. Its initiators see it as based on a guiding style that helps patients say why and how they might change, giving the patient control over the what, why, and how of change and not tricking them into doing what providers want. Specific guidance for MI may be found in Rollnick, Butler, Kinnersley, Gregory, and Mash (2010). A summary of studies of MI embedded in standard diabetic care found mixed results and concluded that such practice was premature, as it did not offer advantages over usual care. It may be that MI's application to chronic disease is different from addiction, on which it was developed (Heinrich, Candel, Schaper, & de Vries, 2010).

IDENTITY AND HOW TO BALANCE CULTURAL AND MEDICAL VALIDITY

Like approaches to motivation, health care's attitude toward personal identity is influential in helping patients achieve SM skills. The mantra of evidence-based medicine (EBM) equates autonomy with treatment choice, in general meaning that patients select their preferences from a predetermined list rather than helping patients engage in meaningful reflection on how available treatment options will affect their lives and goals. In this light, EBM is ultimately physician-centric (Bluhm, 2009), in that a moral meaning to personal identity involves a constructed narrative that demonstrates intentionality, reasoned choice, and coherence (Bok, Mathews, & Rabins, 2009).

Inappropriately practiced, PSM may bind a patient's identity to the language and logic of the disease he or she is managing, demanding compliance with its current medical treatment and blaming the patient if it doesn't yield standard biological markers. Practiced in this way, PSM can alter the patient's former person and diminish patient freedom. Well practiced support should integrate PSM into the patient's identity, admitting alternate kinds of authority other than the "scientific" truths on which medical treatments are thought to be based.

An example may be found in analysis of the rhetoric of patient self-empowerment in depression. Such rhetoric is highly gendered, equating women's emotional states to illness. Advertisements for antidepressants invoke a strong sense of culpability for individuals who fail to seek pharmaceutical interventions, painting this decision as a careless and selfish act against one's social network. In addition, the rhetoric binds the illness of depression to moods and common affective experiences, ensuring that the boundaries of health are never entirely clear and heightening anxieties about how to interpret whether one is ill. In this context, it is possible for the illness to become one's identity (Emmons, 2010).

Patient empowerment can be misused by pharmaceutical marketing that supports self-diagnosis of contested disease states and prescribes outcomes favorable to the company's drug. In this way, disease marketing can transform the identity of a patient who has medical needs into a consumer with culturally significant desires to take control of his or her health. Disease is commercialized and self-diagnosis becomes a pharmaceutically shaped marketing tool, deceiving patients into thinking they are being empowered to demand a diagnosis that requires the company's product (Ebeling, 2011).

Learning is essential to making the transition in identity, not only in adjusting to the chronic disease but also in further development of basic capabilities. A study of individuals with two months of experience in learning to live with diabetes found them focused on listening to and understanding and prioritizing the different body signals. This attentiveness created motivation to change habits toward a new, healthier life. Participants exposed themselves to different situations either to maintain their earlier life or to achieve new experiences in learning how to live with the illness (Kneck, Klang, & Faberberg, 2011).

One destructive factor that can accompany chronic disease and may be avoided or fed by health professionals is stigma. Especially evident with neurological disease and mental health issues, stigma accompanies many chronic diseases, based on the belief that an individual could have prevented the disease by avoiding lifestyle risks (e.g., related to COPD or AIDS), or is dirty and diseased. Stigma can be self-created (internalized), experiential (sometimes from health professionals), or anticipated and has a negative effect on identity and quality of life. Those who anticipate greater stigma from health workers will often avoid accessing health care. Because more than half of adults are living with at least one chronic illness, stigma, social devaluation, or discrediting due to their illness or being denied care or receiving poor care are all potential harms (Earnshaw & Quinn, in press).

Indeed, participants with bipolar disease considered internalized stigma to be a factor that significantly affected their ability to self-manage, adding the necessity of reclaiming their identity and recovering their roles in society. These individuals faced a constant negotiation between the stereotype-laden social identity and the self-identity they chose to adopt. Individuals with a concealable stigma such as manifestations of mental illness have a choice of whether to disclose their condition to others, a choice which in itself can be distressing. But well-functioning persons with bipolar disease were found to have rejected stigma and the isolation that can accompany it, and through actively managing stigma in addition to managing their disease did not internalize it (Michalak et al., 2011).

A common developmental transition from childhood to adolescence and then to adulthood involves a continuum to self-managed care. An example may be found in children receiving liver transplants who display nonadherence with a medical regimen that has a good evidence base supporting its necessity. A study suggests those transplanted at a young age display more difficulty with their transition journey because their identity is more likely to be merged with the disease; in addition, the children appear to be at greater risk of cognitive deficits that could undermine SM. A Developmentally Based Skills Checklist for pediatric liver transplant patients describes necessary SM behaviors, with norms for children less than age ten and those age ten and above; the checklist may be found in Piering et al. (2011).

A different sociocultural dynamic has been described for understanding high risk behavior among nondominant minorities. Labeled a social resistance framework, it argues that power relations in society encourage some members of these groups to actively engage in unhealthy behaviors, resulting in higher rates of mortality and morbidity relative to the majority group. The framework suggests that as a result of discrimination, these individuals may feel alienation, which leads to defying the dominant group along with strong group pressures not to be seen as "acting white." Agency theories suggest that people make "bad choices" in reaction to the conditions in which they live. Resistance theory suggests that frustration due to perceived subordination and the resulting humiliation and anger overrides awareness of hazards and is a means of expressing distrust of professionals and reconstitution of rules. Engaging in health investment behavior (abstaining from smoking or drinking) may be viewed as buying into the dominant and paternalistic narrative (Factor, Kawachi, & Williams, 2011).

Such a pattern was described among some African Americans who did not have their blood pressure controlled. Although participants in this study understood the behaviors necessary to prevent hypertension and believed that following guidelines was important, their commitment to doing so was strongly influenced by intergenerational culture about diet and trust in physicians. This commitment to shun "acting white" created tension between doing what they knew was best for their health versus risking disharmony with the group (Peters, Aroian, & Flack, 2006). A strong message for PSM programs is to fully incorporate nondominant minority leadership and to empower communities to make them heard by the dominant group (Factor et al., 2011).

IMPORTANCE OF DIGNITY

In helping patients learn to self-manage, health care professionals are obliged to consider the role of dignity. Although its definition is controversial, the importance of dignity as expression of respect for persons is not. If dignity means living according to one's principles, violation of dignity involves indifference, condescension, dismissal, and disregard. Such violations cause injury to self-respect, confidence, and a sense of one's self as valuable, worthy, and good; furthermore, such violation is an affront to moral agency (beliefs, standards). These conditions are tied to social orders in which multiple forms of inequity flourish. Instead, PSM should create dignity where it's lacking and maintain dignity where it appears fragile (Jacobson, 2009).

Undoubtedly, health care systems do much to sustain dignity of patients and providers. But systems also have built in pressures that violate dignity, causing breakdown of relationships essential to patient well-being and to providers' ability to care for and attend to what patients are experiencing. Strong patient and family loyalty to caregivers makes dealing with dignity violations difficult. Anger and withdrawal are normal reactions to these violations (Hicks, 2011), causing one to wonder whether they can be one cause of patient noncompliance to regimens. In such a hostile environment patients may not be able to achieve the identity transformation necessary for PSM. Such a journey requires safe and stable relationships in which patient and provider really listen to each other and connect.

MORAL CONFLICTS OF PATIENTS AND FAMILIES

A final component to helping patients build SM skills concerns not just patient choice and decision making, but the wider framework of the person in his or her community. Chronic disease is one of the common calamities that can destroy our sense of control over fate. As accomplished clinicians understand, approaching PSM preparation and support as solely a technical matter denies the moral significance of what the patient is feeling and the need for the patient to develop endurance to accommodate not only life goals and preferences, but also to adjust imagined and ethical aspirations to actual moral experience (Kleinman, 2007). As cultural beliefs and economic patterns indicate, people who are responsible enough to avoid illness, get well (from acute illness), or manage their illness sufficiently will return to work. Persistence of illness due to a chronic state or perhaps because it cannot be controlled adequately enough to allow one to work puts the individual in a deviant role, faced with the moral consequences of not fulfilling one's responsibility for self-support (Walker, 2010).

Also of moral significance are caretaking arrangements, heavily sculpted by cultural assumptions as well as by current world-wide attempts at health care cost containment, which means off-loading care to homes, and from paid employees to health care consumers, therefore reducing labor costs. In our present culture there are no clearly defined limits to the health care burdens that an individual or family group can be expected to take on and no clearly accepted means of exit for those who no longer want to continue caring. Health care work is often elevated as spiritual, moral, or altruistic, yet devalued economically and politically. The role of women in caring work is a sociallycreated arrangement, coerced through cultural norms that daughters, wives, and mothers give care, and is treated as a private versus a public responsibility (Glenn, 2010). This social context denies lay caregivers appropriate professional assistance in the SM they provide.

Ironically, the literature on chronic illness SM among older adults is lacking for minority ethnic groups, the very groups with the highest rates of chronic illness (Gallant, Spitze, & Grove, 2010). But a study of diabetes SM education groups from a multiethnic, socioeconomically deprived London borough showed how PSM can help individuals acquire social meaning and moral worth and rebuild identity through participation in family and community. Stories from participants described the micro-morality of SM choices, balancing economic investment in food, foot apparel, or folk remedies against other life projects and concerns such as providing for the family. Still, economic and moral dimensions are largely absent from official diabetes education materials (Greenhalgh et al., 2011).

The lessons of this chapter for the practice of PSM support might be summarized as follows:

- Beware of inadvertent moral coercion inherent in privileging a health professional point of view and current level of practice that can threaten patients' moral identity as competent people.
- Changing patient beliefs to conform to medical knowledge should be done only when there is a clear benefit to the patient and he or she agrees to do so. Many times "lay" beliefs can coexist with "medical" beliefs, allowing patients to sustain cultural beliefs important to their identities. This chapter has provided several such examples.
- Help patients learn how to detect their irrational reasoning and decisions and how they can be corrected.
- Helping patients develop and sustain a strong sense of confidence (SE) in their ability to carry out all specific skills in their SM regimen is essential.
- Patient autonomy and its effect on identity goes well beyond choosing from a menu of preformed medical disease options. It involves creating options that may not currently exist to meet patient goals. The illness should not become one's identity.
- Give the patient freedom to safely experiment to reach his or her own conclusions about what works and, in the process, to sustain his or her sense of dignity and competence to make the tradeoffs necessary to a sense of what is right.

SUMMARY

Chronic disease and its management, including PSM, precipitate a number of moral questions. Cultural framing of disease and the expectations of caregivers is far from neutral. Attempts to change patient beliefs and motivate them to adopt SM practices can be supportive to capabilities development and positive identity building, or not. One thing is certain—mainstream PSM literature has totally neglected the moral conflicts that patients and families need to address.

STUDY QUESTIONS AND ANSWERS

1. What underlying facts about chronic disease create conditions prone to ethical problems?

   Answer: Perhaps two kinds of facts are most basic: (a) the pattern of progression and accumulation of morbidities, with consideration as to whether they can be slowed or prevented in a particular individual. This fact sets the scene for blaming the victim (the patient didn't comply enough to prevent progression of the disease) and for making standards of practice for health professionals vague; (b) uncertainty and change in the scientific knowledge base by which the disease(s) is(are) managed. Point b is related to a; b means patients must constantly adapt to new scientifically-derived knowledge about which there may be disagreement among providers and that may or may not help them personally and excludes their own observation and experimentation as they are exhorted to "get with" the new evidence. These facts easily undermine their sense of competence in being able to manage their condition. A better strategy is collaborative testing by provider and patient of both evidence-based and patient-derived approaches.

2. Some countries (like the United States) have inequality built into their social policies/institutions. Against such a background, is it possible to reach an appropriate standard of care with poor patients with low levels of education, in order to control their chronic disease?

   Answer: It's a struggle. The first thing to do is not fall into the trap of assuming these patients can't be competent self-managers—in fact, they need SM skills more than other patients because they're likely to have access only to fragmented episodes of care. In the United States, it is possible to help these patients access insurance for which they qualify and a primary care setting in which they can get some continuity of care. More difficult are the social circumstances in which these individuals live, which frequently block access to nutritious food and safe exercise.

3. When symptoms such as long-term pain seem hopeless, patients fail to integrate their illness into their lives, feel deserted and suffer, and find it difficult to take control. Why or how is this an ethical problem?

Answer: Health care and PSM preparation and support should provide tools to help the patient accomplish this task, even if no medical resolution is known. Abandonment is not the answer. A reasonable patient/provider trial entails continuous evaluation of assessment beliefs and changing, on the part of both parties, those that constrain resolution. Beliefs often influence how people experience illness (Jaremo & Arman, 2011).

4. Morality is lived through practices of responsibility, and a story is the basic form to represent a moral problem and construct a moral identity (Porz, Landeweer, & Widdershoven, 2011). Why are stories of responsibility (and therefore moral demands) important in chronic disease?

Answer: Chronic disease is long-standing and ultimately unresolvable, requiring adaptation, and therefore creates a story of struggles which only the individual can make (responsibility). Listening to such a story reveals values, conflicts, and feelings of responsibility.

5. Approximately half of adults who begin a new therapy for chronic disease become nonpersistent in the first year of therapy. Past adherence interventions have largely focused on practical barriers such as forgetfulness or lack of knowledge. Yet, a survey of nearly 20,000 respondents found fear of side effects (especially for diabetes) and lack of perceived need for medication (especially for asthma) were much more frequent than either forgetting to take or inability to afford medications. Clearly, understanding such perceptual barriers in the population being served is essential. What's an ethical principle involved here?

Answer: Patient-centered respect for persons.

6. Should patient informed consent be obtained before PSM preparation?

Answer: Because the point of informed consent is to protect and enable meaningful choice (Beauchamp, 2011), the answer should be yes. Since treatment of chronic disease must include PSM, consent for it can be included in disease treatment. The patient should understand the range of choices including PSM and that this package of treatments can change their self-concept and sense of identity, and demand resources. At its heart, informed consent is a moral doctrine although also a legal doctrine (Beauchamp, 2011).

5

Morally Valid Measurement Model for Patient Self-Management Decisions

It is important to start this discussion by acknowledging that the field of measurement focuses largely on the instrumental aspects of patient education and support of Patient Self-Management (PSM) (i.e., "what works") versus moral validity (measurement that satisfies the range of moral concerns), especially in the way instruments privilege the goals of providers. Clinical judgments made largely on the basis of such measures ignore the fact that patients have a right to complex information, no matter what instrumental outcomes the provider has defined as important. As a linked issue, education in general encompasses a pessimistic view of human nature and a sense that people need to be released from inherent weaknesses. Yet education is much broader than instrumental outcomes. It refers to a person's increasing self-realization of the world and of him-/ herself and is concerned with social justice. The current practice of patient education has been totally captured by the medical model, which is relentlessly instrumental and incorporates various pre determined outcomes not open to negotiation (Standish, Smeyers, & Smith, 2007).

It is encouraging that health scientists are gradually incorporating the instrumental outcomes important to patients into measurement approaches. Yet most instruments of knowledge, beliefs, self-efficacy, and PSM skills are in the very early stages of development and frequently focus on diagnosing patient deficits. Still on the horizon are more fully developed instruments that predict a variety of goals important to all stakeholders and that can be used to enhance people's autonomy by treating them as responsible agents (Standish et al., 2007).

In fact, it is not uncommon to come across studies that find patient perspectives about chronic disease wanting when evaluated by the available measurement tools. Such studies are commonly found in the rheumatic diseases (see study questions for other examples). One such investigation of hand osteoarthritis shows that only one-third of patient-relevant concepts were covered by at least one instrument. Psychological consequences, different qualities of pain, leisure activities, and pain-concerning sensations related to activity were missing from the existing instruments. These discrepancies mean that patient-oriented measures such as self-assessment and understanding the effects of treatment are only partially addressed (Stamm et al., 2009).

As noted in Chapter 4, a patient's display of inadequate self-management (SM) can stem from conflicts fundamental to the person's self-identity; in contrast, lacking PSM skills can be simply a matter of education, of happening not to have skills that one could readily acquire (Standish et al., 2007).

That said, fields of professional practice are also expected to operate with generic standards and with the means to determine if benchmarks have been met. Few standards for PSM exist and those that do have been largely process-oriented, specifying that such elements as a written curriculum are present.

THE DECISIONS: PATIENT SELECTION, SAFETY, SHARED DECISION MAKING, AND GOALS MET

We can describe outcomes currently measured in PSM education, practice, and research in these categories: knowledge, behavior, clinical outcomes, symptom experience, quality of life, attitudes, satisfaction, costs of care, and patient empowerment (Leino-Kilpi, 2011). Several of these taxonomies reflect shared decision making and patient choice, which are so important in chronic disease but represent a significant change in the culture of medicine. What does this changed practice look like and how are its ethical challenges reflected in measurement?

Holm' and Davies's (2009) analysis of these questions is insightful and basic to future development of patient capabilities. Shared decision making, for example, involves exploring patient values with the provider in an advisory role, avoids framing a particular choice as the "right one," and understands that medically preferred care may not be best for the patient as a person or reflect the patient's sense of the interests of his or her family and community. Most quality of life scales measure only health quality and do not reflect a broader, more general quality of life as impacted by health matters (Holm & Davies, 2009).

In spite of these efforts toward a democratized patient-provider relationship, the switch from traditional care has been difficult to accomplish. Yen et al.'s (2011) insightful study of provider reactions to patient perceptions of health issues in chronic illness (often called long-term conditions) is highly instructive. Health professionals often saw the patient experience as either a series of failures related to noncompliance, exacerbated by seeking help inappropriately and poor health literacy, or as a moral issue stemming from patients' failure to make good choices, or as glitches with service fragmentation. Health providers thought these problems should be resolved with additional resources to support providers' activities. Patients, on the other hand, focused on economic hardship, competing demands, and feelings of lack of control in managing co-morbid conditions as criteria for their compliance. Physicians were frustrated when other nonmedical professionals gave patients alternative information, and they resented the need to spend "unpaid time" trying to overcome barriers. Conversely, other professionals were angry that patient access to PSM support services was controlled by physicians, and there was persistent blame shifting for failures. Table 5.1 summarizes these concerns (Yen et al., 2011).

As seen in Table 5.1, health professionals largely agreed with patients on the problems that people with chronic illness face (Yen et al., 2011); on the other hand, cultures, attitudes, and systems entrenched within the medical community led to a dysfunctional situation.

As some indication of progress toward moral validity, a highly relevant use of measurement, the pay-for-performance (P4P), is embedded in incentives meant to reward quality of care. These statistics are also used for public reporting of physician and organizational performance. Two studies from the United Kingdom demonstrate the potential of such systems in diabetes care, along with specific concerns. P4P initiatives provided financial incentives for physicians whose patients reached treatment targets for HbA1c, blood pressure, and cholesterol.

A problem arises, though, as many P4P programs permit physicians to exclude patients from these performance indicators. In a study of 23 general practices in an economically deprived, ethnically diverse part of England, exclusion rates were higher among older patients, ethnic minorities, and those with longer duration of illness, groups that have been shown to experience worse risk factor control and health outcomes (Dalton, Alshamsan, Majeed, & Millett, 2011). Another U.K. study (Millett, Netuveli, Saxena, & Majeed, 2009) found overall improvements in diabetes care indicators associated with P4P but also widening disparities among ethnic groups. Both studies emphasize the point that P4P programs and the measurements they use should be subject to routine monitoring for possible negative impacts (Dalton et al., 2011; Millett et al., 2009).

TABLE 5.1
Patient Concerns and Health Professional Responses

Patient Concerns	Health Professional Responses
Individual level	
Economic hardship	Poor priority setting
Seen in immediate terms as problems of daily life: budgeting, paying for transport, and financial barriers to access	Cost barriers a proxy for moral failure (a few)
	Shaped by social structures: broader welfare problem (majority)
Managing co-morbid conditions	Compliance failures
Lack of control, competing messages from professionals	Inability or unwillingness of patients to focus on management of conditions
Competing demands	
Personal limitations imposed by living with illness and attempting to maintain a "normal" life	Low health literacy resulting in poor motivation and poor ability to navigate health system
Service level	
Economic hardship	Cost shifting
Fragmentation incurs monetary costs in unnecessary travel expenses, medication changes	Problem of poor infrastructure, cross-sector issues, often outside health system
Managing co-morbid conditions	Communication gaps between professionals and professional organizations
Fragmentation incurs time costs—waiting for multiple appointments	Lack of time causing fragmentation
No streamlining or harmonization of services across conditions	Poor communication between different professional groups
	Weak electronic information storage and exchange
Competing demands	Service fragmentation
Obstacles in navigating health system	Lack of accountability between service groups
Treatment by multiple, poorly communicating individual health professionals	Remuneration systems blocking coordination of care

Source: Adapted from Yen, Gillespie, Rn, Kljakovic, Anne Brien, Jan, & Usherwood (2011), *Health Expectations, 14*, pp. 10–12. Copyright © Blackwell Publishing. Used with permission via Copyright Clearance Center.

MONITORING FOR HARMS AS WELL AS FOR BENEFITS IN PSM MEASUREMENT

Harms are inadequately documented in many areas of research and practice. For PSM of chronic disease, harms can include absence of appropriate education and support for mandatory SM; examples of this negligence include provision of wrong information, not attending to patient preferences, confusing patients so that they don't know what to do, and precipitating undue anxiety. All of these are harms of commission among health professionals.

Measures for constructs related to learning can also produce harm. Health literacy, or an individual's ability to seek, understand, and use health information, is widely recognized as an essential skill for PSM and for patient-centered care. Suboptimal health literacy skills reduce the likelihood of maintaining good health and are associated with increased health care costs. Yet a critical appraisal of nineteen instruments measuring the health literacy construct found they focused on reading comprehension and numeracy and not on the full range of skills described in the above definition. In addition, limited empirical evidence on the instruments' reliability and validity raises uncertainty about their accuracy of measurement for all individuals or for populations at risk—a harm in SM education and support (Jordan, Osborne, & Buchbinder, 2011). In fact, a review of the present literature uncovered no studies that assessed the responsiveness of any health literacy instrument essential to its ability to detect a clinically important change or predict ability to self-manage (Jordan et al., 2011).

As another example of dearth of harms monitoring, although traditionally less used in PSM, instruments to measure regret for patient decisions are entirely congruent with the philosophy of patient-provider shared decision making and a democratic relationship. Regret can be seen as an adverse outcome, but also potentially positive if one can use that regret to learn from past mistakes. There are multiple kinds of regret that can occur simply or in combination with other responses: process regret, such as for failing to seek information on all available options; option regret about the alternative choices; role regret in adopting a passive or an active role; and regret about the outcome of a health issue. A thorough review of ten existing instruments of patient decision-making found them unable to capture the various kinds of regret; all instruments assumed negative outcomes for anything approaching this sensibility, and were furthermore rarely used in longitudinal research and so have not described temporal aspects of regret (Joseph-Williams, Edwards, & Elwyn, 2011).

But such rigorous assessment of instruments in a variety of domains relevant to PSM of chronic diseases should be undertaken. From these two examples it is easy to see how findings in a field of clinical practice and/or research can be biased by narrow conceptualization of domains (a form of content or construct validity) as well as by other kinds of errors.

MANDATORY RANGE OF INSTRUMENTS PSYCHOMETRICALLY VALIDATED FOR SM

Examples of PSM instrumentation thus far show that the stable of measurement tools available for assessing patient needs and evaluating outcomes of PSM support programs must be comprehensive for both inclusion of perspectives and the ability to predict important outcomes. Obviously, a set of instruments can be biased in a number of ways; for instance, toward provider-defined outcomes; or by privileging those with middle-class lifestyles, resources, and educational development; or by requiring professional verification.

One kind of instrument to meet PSM goals would capture patient beliefs as valid data. Given the ability of patient beliefs and perceptions to predict their actions (as documented in Chapter 2), measurement of the gap between professional and patient beliefs seems useful. The CONNECT instrument can be used as part of the medical history, assessing perceptions in six domains: The patient's health condition has a biological cause, the patient is responsible for the condition, the patient can control the condition, the condition can be treated by nonbiomedical treatments, the condition has significant meaning for the patient, and the patient prefers a partnership with the physician in managing the condition. Street and Haidet (2011) found that physicians thought their patients' health beliefs were more aligned with their own; however, the physicians' perceptions of patients' health beliefs differed significantly from the actual patient beliefs. In contrast, patients commonly believed they were at fault for any variance from their physicians' understanding and also saw value in natural remedies.

Also useful are instruments that patients can use independently, such as an evidence-based SM urinary incontinence risk factor modification tool designed for older women. In particular, risk factors for urinary incontinence include pelvic floor muscle strength (as well as caffeine intake), as women who correctly perform exercises to strengthen these muscles are 23 times more likely to report symptom improvement than are women who do not use them. The tool was designed for use without formal instruction and was considered successful if a study participant attempted to modify one or more risk factors, and also successful as judged by a decrease in urinary-leakage, self-efficacy, and quality of life. Many women prefer to self-manage their incontinence. The tool requires self-monitoring and so reinforces PSM. Results were comparable to those in pharmacologic trials (Holroyd-Leduc et al., 2011).

Aside from these trends, most measurement instruments are interpreted according to population norms and thus may not represent goals or performance important to individual patients. Goal attainment scaling (GAS) avoids this issue by creating individualized scales of achievement for each patient according to his or her own goals, and then transforming the level of performance into a standard score. For example, persons with chronic low back pain often utilize SM tasks in activities of daily living (ability to wash, dress, move from one position to another), ability to participate in work, and social activities. In short, patients develop and prioritize goals in these or other domains. In addition to the individualization available in this approach, in and of themselves goals can enhance self-engagement and motivation (Mullis & Hay, 2010).

Along with GAS, the strategy of patient identification of a minimally important difference (MID) determines the point in each goal scale that defines the minimum amount of progress the patient feels is needed to significantly improve his or her initial state (Mullis & Hay, 2010). This individualization available through GAS and MID approaches is ethically important.

Much can be done to make instruments and interpretations of their scores more useful. For example, dyspnea management is important for patients with COPD. The Dyspnea Management Questionnaire (Exhibit 5.1) measures multiple dimensions of dyspnea—dyspnea intensity, dyspnea anxiety, activity avoidance, and activity self-efficacy. Its multidimensionality is needed to better measure effectiveness of pharmacologic, pulmonary rehabilitation, and psychosocial interventions (including PSM support) in alleviating both the somatic sensation of dyspnea but also reducing dysfunctional emotions cognitions and behaviors associated with this symptom, that is, highly prevalent in anxious patients. While dyspnea is a modifiable symptom of COPD, research and practice have focused predominantly on evaluating and treating its sensory component. Patients who are helped to understand their responses to all four dimensions of dyspnea are better able to self-manage (Norweg et al., 2011).

Physiologic outcome measures used universally, such as HbA1c for persons with diabetes, can be very limited and should not be used as the sole measure of PSM. Because symptom relief for frequent urination, genital itching, and unintended weight loss may not occur even when HbA1c

EXHIBIT 5.1
DMQ-CAT Items

This questionnaire asks about your breathing and how it has affected your life during the past 2 weeks. We are interested to know how short of breath you have been, how you have been feeling, what activities you may have avoided, and your confidence with managing your breathing difficulty. We will start by asking you four background questions about your gender, use of supplemental oxygen, age, and feelings when short of breath. If you have not performed a particular activity in the last two weeks, give your best estimate of how much shortness of breath you would have had if you had performed the activity. If you have never done a certain activity in your life, rate the question as "not relevant."

I. Dyspnea Intensity
   How short of breath were you in the last 2 weeks while . . .
   1. Showering
   2. Bending down (e.g., picking items up off the floor)
   3. Walking outdoors for one block (1/20 mile) on level ground
   4. Taking out the garbage
   5. Carrying something weighing 10 pounds a distance of 40 feet (such as 2 bags of potatoes or a can of paint)
   6. Climbing one flight of stairs (about 12 steps) without stopping
   7. Carrying a load of wash up a flight of stairs (about 12 steps)
   8. Playing moderate sports such as golf or bowling
   9. Walking 5 miles on level ground
   10. Lifting and carrying furniture such as a 20-pound dining chair 10 feet
   11. Talking and walking with another person

   Not at all short of breath (6)
   Very slightly short of breath (5)
   A little short of breath (4)
   Quite a bit short of breath (3)
   Very much short of breath (2)
   Extremely short of breath (1)
   Not relevant (9)

II. Dyspnea Anxiety
   a)
      1. How upset did you feel during breathing difficulty in the last 2 weeks?
      2. How concerned did you feel during breathing difficulty in the last 2 weeks?

EXHIBIT 5.1
DMQ-CAT Items *(continued)*

3. How much did your breathing difficulty cause you to feel tense in the last 2 weeks?
Not at all (6)
Very slightly (5)
A little (4)
Quite a bit (3)
Very (2)
Extremely (1)

b) How often did you feel . . . during breathing difficulty in the last 2 weeks?
   4. Afraid that you were dying
   5. Worried that something was seriously wrong with you
   6. Afraid of not being able to breathe at all
   7. Your heart was suddenly pounding or racing
   8. Sweaty
Never (6)
Very rarely (5)
Occasionally (4)
Frequently (3)
Almost all the time (2)
All the time (1)

c) How often in the last 2 weeks did you feel . . .?
   9. Worried about a future breathing attack
   10. Bothered by unwanted or distressing thoughts about your breathing difficulty
   11. Your breathing difficulty was out of control
   12. It was hard to concentrate because of your breathing difficulty

III. Activity Avoidance (Example Items)
   How much did you avoid . . . because of breathing difficulty in the last 2 weeks?
   1. Walking uphill for one block (1/20 mile)
   2. Climbing stairs
   3. Visiting friends or family in their home
   4. Doing yard work
   5. Engaging in sexual activities
   6. Doing grocery shopping in a supermarket
   7. Running for short distances
   8. Using public transportation (for example, a bus or a train)

   Did not avoid it at all (6)
   Very slightly avoided it (5)
   Avoided it a little (4)

(continued)

EXHIBIT 5.1
DMQ-CAT Items *(continued)*

Avoided it quite a bit (3)
Avoided it a lot (2)
Completely avoided it (1)
Not relevant (9)

IV. Activity Self-Efficacy (Example Items)
How confident are you to manage breathing difficulty when . . .?
1. Getting dressed
2. Reaching into cabinets and closets above your head
3. Taking out the garbage
4. Climbing one flight of stairs (about 12 steps)
5. Walking inside a mall
6. Sleeping at night
7. Walking for exercise
8. Having a disagreement that upsets you

Extremely confident (6)
Very confident (5)
Quite a bit confident (4)
A little confident (3)
Hardly at all confident (2)
Not at all confident (1)
Not relevant (9)

Source: Adapted from Norweg, Ni, Garschick, O'Connor, Wilke, & Jette (2011),
Archives of Physical Medicine and Rehabilitation, 92, pp. 1561–1567. Copyright
© American Congress of Rehabilitation Medicine. Used with permission of
W. B. Saunders Co. via Copyright Clearance Center.

is at its lowest level, patient self-rated health will be low. With normal
HbA1c readings, almost half of the patients reported typical hyperglycemic symptoms, and patients with different HbA1c levels may report
identical types of symptoms. Both symptoms and self-rated health provide
important additional information (Nielsen, Gannik, Siersma, & Olivarius
Nde, 2011) and should be addressed in PSM education and support.

EXAMPLE OF MEASUREMENT TOOL DEVELOPMENT
IN HEART FAILURE PSM AND OTHERS

Skills needed by patients to perform heart failure SM necessary to maintain
physiologic homeostasis and prevent exacerbations are listed in Table 5.2.

TABLE 5.2
Skills Needed by Patients to Perform Heart Failure Self-Care

Self-care category	Specific skills needed by patients
Maintenance	How to obtain a reliable measure of body weight that can be compared over time
	How to assess one's own ankles for swelling, taking into account the patient's flexibility, body weight, age, blood pressure, and availability of assistance
	How to assess one's fatigue or shortness of breath
	How to read food labels
	How to compensate for coveted high-salt foods in the diet
	How to prepare low-salt foods (note: substitution, portions, alternative cooking methods)
	How to follow a fluid restriction
	How to build a program of physical activity
	How to decide when to forego physical activity based on signs and symptoms
	How to avoid getting ill
	How to talk to your doctor
	How to compensate if a medication dose is missed
	How to order low-salt foods in a restaurant
Management	How to manage a complex medication regimen
	How to differentiate heart failure symptoms from those of other illnesses (specific to a patient's other illnesses)
	How to judge how much liquid to drink on a given day, based on the ambient temperature
	How to decide whether or not to take an extra diuretic dose
	How to know if the treatment was effective

Table 5.2 shows skills that develop over time, fundamental to platforms of PSM (Dickson & Riegel, 2009). Through cumulative work of Barbara Riegel et al. (2011) in testing and improving the psychometric qualities of the Self-Care of Heart Failure Index (SCHFI), stakeholders can accurately measure patients' ability to practice PSM. Those who practice above-average PSM have event-free survival benefits that are much better than those with below-average PSM practices. In Dickson and Riegel's (2009) work, this translated into a 56% reduction of all-cause mortality, hospitalization, or emergency department admission. The index asks patients to report if in the past 3 months they had trouble breathing or ankle swelling, how quickly they recognized either of these as a symptom of heart failure, what they did about it, and their degree of confidence that the remedy helped. Further research has identified patients who have not yet become physically limited by heart failure and who have a low symptom burden, still feel in control, and are not motivated to engage actively in SM. These patients are inconsistent in their self-monitoring practices and may need extra assistance in developing SM expertise (Riegel et al., 2011). But further research has noted that symptomatic heart failure patients who practice above-average PSM have an event-free survival benefit similar to that of symptom-free heart failure patients (Lee, Moser, Lennie, & Riegel, 2011).

An instrument with this level of predictive validity is rare but ought to be available for all chronic diseases. Although not as well developed psychometrically, two other examples of instruments illustrate true patient focus. In the first, age-related macular degeneration is a leading cause of impaired vision with which many elderly individuals cope. Rovner et al. (2011) describe an outcome measure of targeted vision function, referring to specific vision-dependent goals patients highly value but find difficult to achieve. An intervention that teaches problem solving around those goals supports the outcome measure, surely more patient-relevant than simply a measure of vision.

A second example addresses the notion of self-efficacy, commonly regarded as predictive of a person's taking a particular action. Measures of self-efficacy in condom use and HIV medication adherence have been developed. But in this example, instead of measuring a compliance-like action, the HIV Symptom Management Self-Efficacy for Women Scale measures patient self-efficacy beliefs about managing the symptoms of HIV/AIDS. Although detection of symptom changes and learning how to treat them, communicate with health care providers, and self-intervene to control symptom changes over time are complex tasks, they actually lessen the burden of self-managing chronic illnesses associated with HIV/AIDS (Webel & Okonsky, 2011). The relevance to PSM of this new measure on symptom management is that it is patient-centered and should be applied during the time the patient is learning this complex new set of behaviors.

A final illustrative example of the state of measurement can be found in a consensus report on the role of self-monitoring of blood glucose in non-insulin treated type 2 diabetes (Klonoff et al., 2011). This practice is well-established for patients with type 1 diabetes mellitus and for insulin-treated persons with type 2 diabetes mellitus but uncertain for those not treated with insulin. Its potential benefits include: preventing, identifying and treating hypoglycemia; providing feedback on the results of lifestyle and pharmacologic treatments; providing information for both patient and provider to inform treatment modifications and titrations; and increasing patient empowerment by understanding what factors affect their glycemic levels and how to modify those factors. But the value of a measurement (which has been "did the patient do blood glucose self-monitoring [BGSM]") is dependent on how the data were used and here is the weakness. Patients and providers require education on how to respond to data—when and how frequently should BGSM be performed, and what is the meaning of various BG levels and how can that information be used?

Self-management blood glucose [SMBG] targets must be individualized, especially for patients at risk for hyperglycemic and hypoglycemic events. Patients have frequently not been encouraged to adjust treatment based on SMBG values, although new software will instruct on what type of action to take based on pre-programmed individual factors and real-time blood glucose [BG] data. Few patients have a thorough understanding of how to react to abnormal results; a structured educational program is necessary to achieve these results. SMBG can also provide data on end points other than A1c, such as hypoglycemic events very meaningful to patients.

The lesson in this example is the disconnect between a measure of patients doing BGSM and changes in the end state—A1c or hypoglycemic episodes—and the fact that data might be collected and never acted upon because patients (and maybe providers) don't know what to do with it.

SUMMARY

The quality of measurement in health care is critically important for at least two reasons. First, in order to develop guiding standards and work toward improvement, high quality measures must be established well enough to have the confidence of clinicians. Because PSM is central to managing most chronic diseases, which vary in the tasks and judgments required of the patient, a number of such instruments are called for. Currently, only the SCHFI for cardiac failure reaches the level of psychometric validity required; Riegel and colleagues' (2011) program of research serves as a model of the development that must happen in other fields of PSM.

Health care today still lacks valid measures to monitor most chronic diseases (Pronovost, Marsteller, & Goeschel, 2011). We owe our patients higher levels of quality. Furthermore, biases in measurement are common, and frequently in PSM reflect the position of compliance with medical regimens and confound the quality of medical management and PSM. Both deficient quality and bias are moral issues.

In the United States, the Affordable Care Act established the Patient-Centered Outcomes Research Institute (PCORI) to respond to a widespread concern that patients, families and caregivers do not have the information they need to make choices aligned with the health outcomes they desire. PCORI is an independent, nonprofit private entity with a goal of supporting study designs and outcomes relevant to people making choices, addressing questions such as *What are my options (benefits and harms?)* And *What can I do to improve outcomes most important to me?* (Washington & Lipstein, 2011).

STUDY QUESTIONS AND ANSWERS

1. Chronic pain accompanies some chronic diseases and must be self-managed. A large-scale survey of people with chronic pain found a more extensive range of treatment outcomes rated important than are frequently used in trials. Some outcomes noted by patients as important, such as difficulty concentrating and difficulty remembering things, were not assessed in any of the 60 trials reviewed. So, while patient-reported outcomes are now a required component of evaluation and audit, outcomes measured are usually those determined important by clinicians and researchers rather than those determined by patients. Assuming that range of measures is at least as important as is psychometric quality, how would you balance these two characteristics? What is the ethical issue here?

   Answer: Range and psychometric quality are both important. The ethical issue goes directly to the notion of validity. Decisions made on the basis of a limited range of measured outcomes fail to recognize patient priorities and values and therefore undermine their agency.

2. Clinical trials in rheumatoid arthritis (RA) currently focus on measuring severity of functional disability, patient global assessment, pain, and morning stiffness. But inclusion of patient-reported outcomes and collaboration with patients to develop outcome measures are mandatory. Such collaborations have identified three aspects of impact: severity of an outcome, its importance to the patient, and the patient's ability to self-manage. For example, focus group data exploring patient definition of flare in RA identified these factors and found especially important from the patient's view that actions they took to deal with the flare failed (SM), requiring seeking medical help. So, a patient's model of flare goes beyond a simple increase in number of swollen joints or intensity of pain (Sanderson et al., 2011). What is likely to be the effect of including questions regarding patients' perceived ability to self-manage symptoms?

   Answer: Such a move should increase patient safety because it acknowledges patient ability to self-manage as important and measures it, triggering need for better SM education and support or documenting lack thereof.

3. Instruments to structure patient self-risk assessment are being developed and tested. For example, albuminuria is a key subclinical marker for kidney disease. There is a treatment for it, yet routine screening for high risk patients does not reliably occur. A self-assessment tool of risk factors (age; race; sex; current smoking; self-rated health; and self-reported history of diabetes, hypertension and stroke) can be completed by an individual at home or in settings like health fairs. Based on the score, individuals with high priority of albuminuria can request screening. This tool still needs external validation (Muntner et al., 2011). Thus SM can involve not only monitoring and interventions but also widespread public risk assessment at preclinical stages of chronic disease. Is that problematic?

Answer: On balance, probably not. Although it has the potential to increase surveillance, which might be experienced as invasive, such risk assessment is one more tool patients can use to fill the gaps in appropriate clinical and population-based health programs.

4. Outcome Measures in Rheumatology Clinical Trials (OMERACT) has worked over the years to achieve consensus on core sets of outcome measures in rheumatologic diseases, with a strong focus on patient-reported outcomes. Outcome has been defined as how a patient feels, functions, and survives. Persons with RA mentioned fatigue as one of their most bothersome symptoms, although it was not included in the agreed core measures for RA clinical trials. International consensus was reached that fatigue should be measured in all RA studies using a validated instrument (Tugwell et al., 2011). What is the ethical issue here?

Answer: The first thing to note is that OMERACT is making a serious sustained effort to create standards that reflect patient views about effective treatment. To this author's knowledge, OMERACT's efforts are by far the most advanced of any disease entity. The measurement concept "validity" does require that all relevant domains be included, and fatigue obviously hasn't been, probably because patients weren't asked. Knowing this, PSM programs should include ways to self-mange this symptom and use measures to assess their effectiveness. Like any other program, PSM should aim to optimize benefits to patients and respect their ability to identify what their needs are.

5. A person's health literacy (ability to seek, understand, and use health information) is critical to active participation in health care. Current health literacy screening instruments measure reading and ability to recognize words. Patients, however, describe literacy much more broadly to include knowing when and where to seek health information; capacity to process, retain, and use information; and change health information with health professionals (Jordan et al., 2011). Is this mismatch of concern?

Answer: Yes, because current instruments misdiagnose (or likely underdiagnose) literacy problems. The lesson learned is to involve patients in definition of a domain before constructing a measurement instrument.

6. Much research on patient compliance (adherence) with medical regimens (especially with medications) has focused on various means by which to get an accurate account of how much of the prescribed regimen the patient has taken. Much less frequently do we measure the reasons for noncompliance, which means that interventions used are not explicitly matched to reasons for non-adherence. Reasons can include patients thinking medications are not needed, and/or the regimen is too complex to understand or carry out, and/or lack of resources to obtain a prescription to buy medications and/or mistaking symptom remission as healing of the disease. Indeed, a patient can be adherent with one medication but non-adherent with another. What's the ethical effect of measuring rate of compliance and not measuring reasons for it?

Answer: Blaming the patient and not moving to more useful measurement strategies.

7. Business leaders describe very basic errors in understanding cost of health care for a particular patient—costs are allocated not based on actual resources used to deliver care, but on how much they are reimbursed. There is almost complete lack of understanding of how much it costs to deliver patient care, much less how those costs compare with outcomes achieved. Better measurement of outcomes will lead to significant improvements in the value of health care delivered, as providers' incentives shift away from performing highly reimbursed services and toward improving the health status of patients

(Kaplan & Porter, 2011). What is the relevance of this situation for PSM of chronic disease?

Answer: First, since PSM education and support have not historically been reimbursed, providers have a disincentive to provide it. Second, because measurement has been so badly done, no one has any idea how much it costs to support PSM, including potential offsets from reduction in provider services, or of the value added. Third, costs and value are not transparent to patients to help them decide what they want to purchase. Measuring the wrong thing is disastrous, but doing so on a grand scale is not that unusual and is a serious ethical problem.

6

Technologies in Patient Self-Management

We are familiar with the evolution of technology in health care for disease management; it serves similarly in patient self-management (PSM). But at the same time that technology enables PSM, it also poses a series of ethical questions: Is it safe and easy to use? Does it enable learning and capability building? Does it invade privacy? Does it structure the patient's existence so as to rule out valued activities and identities? Technology clearly changes expectations for the patient's role in managing chronic disease. PSM supportive technologies may be arbitrarily divided into categories of electronic or digital and those that utilize home-based equipment (but these may overlap, of course). Finally, PSM could itself be regarded as social innovation with embedded technologies; in this chapter we consider how it might evolve and how to address its vulnerabilities.

INFORMATION HEALTH TECHNOLOGIES AND PSM SUPPORT SYSTEMS

Online therapies, personal health records (PHRs), interactive web sites and iPhones are digital technologies that have been adapted for PSM training/support. Additionally, Telehealth care (also known as Telecare), an integrated support system, installs services in patients' homes to monitor predefined risk parameters (Mathar, 2011). Although private companies are usually involved in commercializing these products and services (frequently with little oversight), digital technologies offer greatly expanded training opportunities for patients in widely dispersed geographical sites, as well as the opportunity to learn complex decision making required for many chronic diseases and the safe management of chronic diseases at home.

Online therapies such as awareness training for blood glucose level, depression, and other conditions, developed using cognitive behavioral theory, are cheaply available and can reach millions. Safeguards include patient use of a screening questionnaire that can indicate need of emergency care or deem the patient unlikely to benefit from the current treatment offered. Another safety net involves patient completion of modules checked by questionnaires to gauge progress and provide personalized feedback, ranging from no medical intervention needed to recommending a therapist or psychologist stay in frequent e-mail or phone contact with the patient (Nowak, 2008).

More complex therapies are adaptable to PSM, too. Diabetic insulin infusion is an example of a therapy that frequently requires 2 to 4 months of educational support before the patient has mastered both the pump and advanced self-management (SM) skills such as basal rates and programs, bolus doses and presets, and insulin correction and adjustment. Traditionally, insulin pump manufacturers have been the primary source of information about their devices through marketing materials or user manuals. Following this trend, Sirotinin (a full-time employee of the company) developed an interactive training CD that allows patients to practice pump operation and provides corrective feedback to help them better understand and manage their diabetes (Sirotinin & George, 2010). As useful as these promotional materials appear, however, we should remember their prime purpose is to sell the product.

Electronic PHRs can be designed with PSM supports such as storage and charting of health indicators (e.g., blood pressure [BP] readings), confirmation of medication lists, decision aids, reminders, tailored instruction, even motivational feedback; in addition, the PHR can link to credible health information online. The National Health Service in the United Kingdom has invested in this application. Interactive web sites are operated in a manner similar to the PHR (Or et al., 2011; Yamin et al., 2011). To date, iPhones have more limited capabilities, but this lag calls for remediation. For persons with diabetes, iPhones should develop the ability to integrate data from blood glucose monitors and convert insulin-to-carbohydrate ratios to insulin dose (Ciemins, Coon, & Sorli, 2010).

As seen here, digital products and services show potential, yet problematic implementation of technology-supported PSM includes limited or no reimbursement to providers for employing it, as well as the familiar "digital divide" in adoption and use of the PHR. A recent study showed that racial/ethnic minority patients and those with lower incomes utilized a PHR less frequently than White patients and those with higher incomes; ironically, the former groups have the greatest potential to experience PSM benefits (Yamin et al., 2011).

A more complete system of connecting technologies, including the use of smart sensors, is known as Telecare. This system provides continuous feedback and instruction and is especially useful for chronically ill persons who live at home but need frequent contact with professional caregivers. However, these patients' wellness aims have not been substantiated, including improved health status and quality of life, diminished number of exacerbations and hospitalizations, and receiving more effective and efficient care. Therefore, we need to ask: How do these systems as currently designed support PSM?

Three degrees of PSM have been defined as: (1) patient takes over practical tasks such as measurement from the health professional, (2) patient learns interpretive and decisional tasks from the professional and then takes action to manage his or her condition, and (3) patient is enabled to find his or her own way of living with the condition, including the ability to enhance quality of life and fulfill important life goals and values. Telecare promotes the first level of PSM but may discourage level 3, which is the most ethically satisfying due to its focus on helping the patient understand how to follow a medical regimen, and also by its collection of data to ensure this occurs (i.e., patient submits monitoring results, documents subsequent action) (Schermer, 2009).

As a last note, electronic technologies have been used in some countries to change the role of patients. Analysis of policy documents in the English Department of Health shows patients viewed as capable and willing to make their own decisions, and as active persons who wish to live independently, monitored by Telehealth. There is a policy theme of "empowering" patients, assuming they are able to take over as many disease-management tasks as possible (Mathar, 2011). We glean from this example that information technologies can cause social disruption by fundamentally changing patterns of communication (Carlsen et al., 2010), in this case among patients, providers and managers of the health care system. Yet, while Telehealth has been demonstrated to produce certain benefits (e.g., timely access to and a sense of relationship with health professionals, as well as a sense of decreased burden of illness), a study of the service found that when used as the sole health care support, it reinforced dependency on health providers and enhanced a perception of the right to use services instead of developing capabilities for supported self-sufficiency (Rogers, Kirk, Gately, May, & Finch, 2011).

Electronic connectivity to patients may, in fact, be an important solution to the vast amount of PSM needed for the rapidly growing number of patients with chronic diseases. It can emphasize PSM with just-in-time provider intervention (which can be motivating, educational, and caring) and can avoid the current limitations of face-to-face encounters between patients and providers at specific locations. In other words, electronic connectivity is a prime tool for developing patient capability for the highest level of SM. Sensors in a wearable patch can measure thoracic impedance (a proxy for fluid congestion in the lungs) for persons with heart failure and can collect continuous physiologic monitoring data, transmitting it through a wireless hub in the home. Households near the poverty line are likely to have only cell phones and, thus, can be better engaged and motivated through this approach. But such applications will not occur without changes in the reimbursement model (Kvedar, Nesbitt, Kvedar, & Darkins, 2011).

HOME, MOBILE, AND PERSONAL TECHNOLOGIES

Home health care devices are used for several purposes; for example, to monitor or diagnose (e.g., International Normalized Ratio [INR] meters, peak flow meters, self-diagnosis kits for urinary tract infection or pregnancy), disease treatment (e.g., infusion pumps, home dialysis machines), and rehabilitation (Bitterman, 2011). In spite of their ubiquity, descriptions of home device use in diabetes, cardiovascular and respiratory conditions illustrate the shaky foundations on which home technologies are sometimes implemented, from poorly conceived studies to lack of attention regarding accuracy of measurement. But studies also portray significant benefits when the technologies are appropriately combined to yield rapid feedback and correction of treatment and patient learning.

As one instance of popular but precarious home device use, blood glucose monitoring machines that allow self-monitoring, based on the theory that optimal insulin coverage requires knowledge of current glycemic level and carbohydrate content of the meal, have now become standard practice, especially in type 1 diabetes, to avoid prolonged periods of high glucose levels and limit risk for hypoglycemic episodes. Yet randomized controlled trials of SM for blood glucose (SMBG) have shown inconsistent results in type 1, type 2, and gestational diabetes. An obvious conceptual error in these trials is to assume that patients who practice SMBG actually do something with the information (Kolb, Kempf, Martin, Stumvoll, & Landgraf, 2010). In fact, a small study (Peel, Douglas, & Lawton, 2007) showed that not only did patients tend not to act on their self-monitoring results, but that continued high readings created a sense of failure among patients that led to abandonment of dietary regimens. Interestingly, no patients reported receiving ongoing education about SMBG.

In another intriguing finding, a cognitive task analysis of PSM in diabetes showed the steps to be very complex, well beyond the simple rules sometimes conveyed to patients. Diabetes PSM requires skill in comprehending and manipulating variables in a complex dynamic system featuring physiologic and environmental disturbances, as taught in other sophisticated fields by computerized simulation (Lippa, Klein, & Shalin, 2008).

Accuracy of SMBG measurement can be problematic. Drugs and substances can interfere with test results (the effects of acetaminophen, for example, have been known since the 1980s), and strips are approved at the manufacturing site rather than in home conditions affected by changes in temperature and humidity. Indeed, patients frequently do not know of the conditions that affect instrument accuracy (Heinemann, 2010). To illustrate, a study showed that a number of home glucose monitors are insufficiently calibrated at low blood glucose levels to accurately detect hypoglycemia. Although there is no consensus in the health care community that the devices are accurate enough to assess hypoglycemia, these monitors are increasingly used by patients to achieve tight glycemic control (Sonmez et al., 2010). But in another field requiring accurate measurement—oral anticoagulation SM—patients were able to learn and incorporate into their practice the external quality assurance measures similar to those used in institutional laboratories (Murray, Jennings, Kitchen, Kitchen, & Fitzmaurice, 2007). Such formal safeguards should be available in all PSM technologies.

Shifting our gaze to a cardiovascular context, home measurement of BP has been established as more predictive of end organ damage than periodic provider measurement. A close analysis of the situation in a random controlled trial revealed that telemonitoring and SM added self-titration of antihypertensive drugs combined with telemonitoring, so that readings made at home were relayed to a health care professional who could take appropriate action. This approach guaranteed that patients were not ignoring very high or low readings. Such a combination of technologies and services yielded better control of BP than what was achieved with usual care and could make a significant contribution to population-based hypertension control, even though the trial excluded patients with more than two hypertension medications (McManus et al., 2010).

New approaches to management of heart failure, such as telemonitoring, are built on the assumption that remote surveillance would detect early decompensation, facilitate early intervention, and decrease hospital readmissions of these patients. But one trial showed no benefit of telemonitoring over usual care. It is important to gain an understanding and resolution of this problem. Perhaps currently used physiologic measures such as weight gain and symptoms are poor surrogates for filling pressures, and therefore are inadequate markers to anticipate the onset of decompensation. Or perhaps, as noted in the diabetes trials above, the responses to information from telemonitoring by patients and professionals were insufficient (Desai & Stevenson, 2010).

The effectiveness of telemedicine in treatment failure is not established; neither is the profile of patients who can potentially benefit from telemedicine in stabilization, crisis prevention, and self-empowerment. Reimbursement strategies are also not in place (Anker, Koehler, & Abraham, 2011). Early detection remains problematic and requires clarity about what combination of changes in agreed variables detects what is abnormal for a particular patient, for a predictive alert. Because it's important to be clear about who is accountable for taking action or for the risk of taking no action, there is need to co-design the technology and the health services collaboratively (Hardisty et al., 2011).

A second trial studying missed detection of heart failure (Soran et al., 2010), which was carried out in primary care practices, compared enhanced patient education (control group) and follow-up with home installation of an electronic scale and an individualized response system linked by phone line to a computerized data base staffed by nurses (experimental group). Randomized to the sophisticated home monitoring treatment, patients were instructed to weigh themselves daily and record heart failure symptoms, and were taught when to contact a health care provider. There were no differences in clinical outcomes between the two groups, and the experimental treatment was more costly. Perhaps in this study and among these patients there was relatively little room left for altering the natural course of the disease, or the primary care physicians didn't respond appropriately to clinical deterioration. At any rate, the quest to find a better way to monitor and manage this expensive disease that leads to poor quality of life continues.

Building on studies that suggest management of ambulatory hemodynamics may improve outcomes in chronic heart failure, a first-in-human study implanted a left atrial pressure monitor with readings acquired twice daily, and more frequently if patients had worsening symptoms. Based on the readings, individualized medication instructions were given to patients to avoid pulmonary congestion. The frequency of elevated left atrial pressure readings was significantly reduced, and there were improvements in New York Heart Association class and left ventricular ejection fractions (Ritzema et al., 2010). This beginning work in ambulatory hemodynamics using patient-administered measurement technologies is one type of exploration for improving the management of heart failure.

Telemonitoring systems for managing heart failure are still evolving in terms of the data collected and how they are managed. Physiologic data (body weight, heart rate, BP, body temperature) or electrocardiogram tracings, oxygen saturation, and physical activity data are noninvasive. Other systems enable transfer of variables measured invasively, including impedance and pulmonary and left arterial pressures. Telemedical home assessment units can measure concentrations of blood chemicals or biomarkers, or monitor function and usage of already implemented devices such as implantable cardioverter-defibrillator (ICD) shocks and pacemakers. Data may be "send and store" or may be analyzed by automatic algorithms, or may even provide constant analytical and decision-making support.

Yet, much is still unknown about these variables—what is the clinically relevant size of change in body weight over what time period? Telemedicine can provide the heart failure patient with a structured disease management process and should be developed to also manage comorbidities and to optimize SM abilities of patients (Anker et al., 2011).

Finally, in respiratory-related health care, proper use of inhalers for both rescue and controller medications is important for persons with asthma and COPD. A study of a predominantly minority hospitalized population with frequent disease exacerbations and a history of near-fatal respiratory events found very high inhaler misuse rates. Although lacking a control group, this study found that with use of a teach-to-goal approach unassociated with health literacy level, all patients learned the appropriate inhaler technique. However, the study also documented problems with technology design and use. Symptom control and prevention of exacerbations often require combination therapy with two or more types of inhalers that may have different and sometimes conflicting instructions for use. In the study, the type size on directions was too small for several patients with vision limitations. As a further complication, there is no consensus on the most appropriate threshold for defining correct versus incorrect use of respiratory inhalers (Press et al., 2011). These home device inadequacies can have serious consequences for patients and, sadly, are preventable with adequate technology design, PSM education, and support.

Fortunately, we see implementation of home technologies improve when founded on a combination of PSM and care monitored by health personnel. Some home health agencies, using home monitoring to detect exacerbations for persons with chronic disease, have designed their programs specifically to launch patient skills for independent PSM once the technology is withdrawn (usually after 3–4 weeks). The program design allows collection and storage of vital sign data, which are forwarded to a secure web site. Telehealth nurses provide real-time education about cause and effect relationships between personal behaviors and the obtained physiological results. But because of lack of reimbursement for remote patient monitoring, this service can be locally and regionally disparate, even though it reduces operating costs of the agency, likely through a diminished need for home visits (Suter, Suter, & Johnston, 2011).

Three points about the ethics of this situation are relevant to technology use in PSM. First, slow or incomplete dissemination of technologies are a prime source of health disparities. Second, technologies for PSM must be developed to meet the needs of disadvantaged patients, particularly those with limited literacy and/or numeracy. Technologies should be developed interactively, taking into account the variety of persons who use them. Third, it is important to note that technologies are designed to preserve certain roles, mostly medical roles. What is the basis for home blood glucose monitoring that allows and directs patients to not only detect abnormalities but treat them, when home BP monitoring allows only detection? Is this because diabetes requires quick correction while hypertension does not, or because the latter correction is more complex and thus not understandable to persons with hypertension? One reasonable alternative answer is that home or personal technologies are designed according to medical beliefs about appropriate roles.

ETHICS IN TECHNOLOGY ASSESSMENT

Such assumptions as outlined above (as well as others) should be built into the formal assessments carried out, often by government agencies, to set standards for technologies, including those for use in the home. These agencies provide recommendations for policy makers about safety and benefits and often become the basis for payment decisions. In situations of moral conflict, ethical analysis should provide a thorough scrutiny and contribute to resolution. Historically, it has been difficult for such agencies to include assessment of value assumptions built into technologies. A recent survey by the International Network of Agencies for Health Technology Assessment revealed disparate methods for making values and ethical issues explicit (Burls et al., 2011). The group developed a framework of questions to help structure considerations of ethical issues by agencies doing technology assessment (TA). These include the following queries:

- Why was this technology selected for assessment? Does it involve all stakeholders in the selection so that industry-driven priorities do not predominate?
- At what point in a technology's development should it be assessed? Technologies assessed too early may appear ineffective while those assessed too late may have become established to an appropriate degree. Technologies deemed effective may not have become adequately diffused into practice.
- Characteristics of this and related technologies are important. TA is always comparative with related technologies that may not have been assessed. A technology may establish responsibilities for users.
- Are there morally relevant issues in choice of endpoints, such as decreased mortality/morbidity, increased functional status, increased quality of life? How are these (and other) endpoints balanced?
- Are there morally relevant issues in the primary studies on which the TA is based? Methodologically weaker study designs may overestimate a technology's effectiveness. Are the users in the studies typical of those that will apply it (i.e., patients and families)?

We should beware of health TAs that focus entirely on scientific objectivity and don't acknowledge that data and methods are inevitably value laden (Burls et al., 2011). (See Chapter 5 for a fuller description of measurement issues.)

So, to summarize, ethics can analyze the consequences of technology implementation and improvements in health decision making but should also investigate and justify the normative structure of the technology and of its assessment. Several methods from ethical analysis can be used and may enlighten different facets of this issue. Casuistry is a form of case-based reasoning that requires consideration of circumstances surrounding an ethical question or issue. The key task in casuistry is to propose cases that are sufficiently similar to the present case in order to warrant the same or a different resolution. For example, the question of whether morbid obesity that warrants bariatric surgery is a disease or a character flaw bears on the question of whether the surgery should be reimbursed or the patient held responsible. Comparable situations can be found in society's response to helping people about to drown (we rescue them) or those attempting suicide (we help them, in spite of the stigma surrounding self-inflicted harm, in the same way that we help people with sports injuries or sexually transmitted disease) (Saarni, Braunack-Mayer, Hofmann, & van der Wilt, 2011).

In a different model flowing from principlism (a theory framework comprised of concern for patient autonomy, beneficence, non maleficence, justice), four criteria for just decisions are need, capacity to benefit, rights, and merit. If candidates for bariatric surgery do not differ in these respects from other patients, then there are no grounds for discriminating against them (Saarni et al., 2011).

SOCIAL NETWORKING

We now turn to the role that technology external to health care plays on PSM. Facebook offers patients an opportunity to build and benefit from a social network to understand others' experiences. Since it is an unregulated environment, it is important to know the extent to which its information is clinically accurate versus biased toward particular products or suggestive of potentially harmful conclusions. A recent study (Greene, Choudhry, Kilabuk, & Shrank, 2011) analyzed discussion topics and wall posts from the fifteen largest Facebook groups focused on diabetes management. Promotional activity and personal data collection were common, and there were no editorial monitors or fact checkers. But to Facebook's credit, the discussions favored patient-centered goals, providing specialized knowledge from peers and allowing participants to articulate their realistic self-images as diabetic individuals.

A study of ten online social network sites on diabetes found that nine featured advertising, including unfounded "cures" on three sites, and only three supported member controls over personal information. PSM support may overlook these dangers because social networking is voluntary and disconnected from institutional authorities. Yet, in this electronic venue several steps could be taken to protect individuals made vulnerable by illness, including periodic external review of member discussions to discover wrong information, clear flagging of commercial content and commercial members, and assurance that privacy policies are easy to find and readable by the majority of health consumers (Weitzman, Cole, Kaci, & Mandl, 2011).

Additional concerns have been raised by Light and McGrath (2010), highlighting lack of transparency about exposure and invasion of privacy among users. For example, a person may believe he or she is merely registering for the system when in reality is creating a profile with personal data and signaling agreement to a default setting that allows a high degree of openness. Users often think of social networking sites as safe and closed worlds. In reality fake profiles can provide a successful cover for cyberstalking and identity theft. Ethical responsibility is very scattered and not well delineated (Light & McGrath, 2010).

The good news is that the electronic era can serve to challenge medical authority and its logic by creating a forum in which the lay view of experience with an illness is magnified and made powerful. Such was the case with breast cancer screening. Medical science has focused on health at the population level, but individuals tend to prioritize medicine's responsibility to provide urgent help to those with a problem. Online forums generate this connectivity among those with a health problem and enhance the moral authority of their claims. Indeed, medical accounts incongruent with lay-people's experiences cause them to create their own coherent accounts and solutions. The Internet has enabled lay expertise to become a collective phenomenon through electronic support groups for nearly every illness (Barker & Galardi, 2011).

PSM AS SOCIAL INNOVATION WITH EMBEDDED TECHNOLOGIES

PSM itself is a disruptive social innovation. It not only changes communication patterns (e.g., disrupting patient-provider dominance) but also can set new performance parameters if PSM education and support and patient actions are documented in electronic records. To assist this advance, all technologies used in PSM should be tested and revised with users and revisited as the innovation changes. And clearly, PSM has already undergone change as more countries center their health policy on this care approach, as seen by patient education becoming more outcome-oriented and longitudinal in its management of chronic disease.

Like every other evolving innovation, however, PSM has weaknesses. Vulnerability analysis identifies such areas in a system, given that weaknesses may limit the system's ability to maintain its intended function when exposed to internal or external threats or hazards (Carlsen et al., 2010). In the case of PSM in health care, what scenarios could be imagined that will guide us in how it evolves?

As another health care advance, a fully developed PSM, along with professional and patient-oriented quality control, could test the limits of our ability to control chronic disease in real life situations. But as chronicled in previous chapters, PSM is currently not consistently available, suffers from lack of quality standards and measures, and is confounded with bias of quality toward medical care. Still, fully professionalizing this approach could allow it to begin meeting what policy makers expect from it—better health outcomes and patient satisfaction at a reasonable cost. If we leave PSM stuck in its current practice, policy makers may well give up on what should be an inevitable new partnership between providers and patients that supports and enables the healthier population central to economic development.

A more reasonable scenario is that health care continues to move from acute care settings to the community. Yet hospitals have been home for much PSM education and support. What community-based institutions are capable of PSM development and long-term coordination of PSM with provider care over the course of chronic disease? In the United States, none immediately come to mind. There is much work to do.

SUMMARY

Technologies that are unfailingly accurate in conditions of daily patient use should be a given. Furthermore, these devices should be simple to learn and remember how to use, as patients may be confused when in physiological crisis states such as high or low blood sugar, or in a state of high emotional agitation as when they need to make critical decisions. Information technologies can be central to PSM but must be understood as disruptive in the way they change patient and provider roles. PSM itself is a social innovation with embedded technologies that will hinder or help its evolution.

STUDY QUESTIONS AND ANSWERS

1. Many PHR systems are physician-oriented, do not include patient-oriented functionalities, and their effectiveness and sustainability for PSM has not been established (Archer, Fevrier-Thomas, Lokker, McKibbon, & Straus, 2011). PHRs are defined as electronic or paper-based collections of health or wellness data managed, controlled or shaped by that individual. What PHR features are essential to its success for patients?

   Answer: Integration with a primary care electronic medical record that can manage communications for prescriptions and appointments; system interoperability to give consumer access to health records in hospital, physician, and lab systems; decision support tools to assist patients in managing chronic illnesses based on monitoring data (including in emergencies) are important (Archer et al., 2011).

2. Devices for home evaluation of colon cancer, breast cancer (simulated breast designed to train women to detect lumps), urinary tract infections, and yeast infections are among detection instruments now available, with new devices for sexually transmitted diseases and strep throat coming to market. The home testing market is booming (Scolaro, Lloyd, & Helms, 2008)—will this be good for patients?

   Answer: It will be advantageous if the tests have been certified as reliable, if results can be kept confidential, and if patients have access to counseling about how to interpret test results and use the information.

3. PSM also includes acute phases of chronic diseases. The research literature is clear that auto-injection of epinephrine (treatment of choice for anaphylactic emergencies) are under-used by patients of all ages. A study of adolescents found confusion about when to use the auto-injector with strong emotional reactions leading to indecision (Gallagher, Worth, Cunningham-Burley, & Sheikh, 2011). What can be done?

   Answer: Revise any teaching program.

4. Although developed for the study of synthetic biology, the Presidential Commission for the Study of Bioethical Issues released principles for assessing emerging technologies. Home- and individual-based technologies supporting PSM of chronic disease can be either individually

or in the aggregate assessed and guided by these principles: public beneficence, responsible stewardship, intellectual freedom and responsible stewardship, intellectual freedom and responsibility, and democratic deliberation, and justice and fairness (Gutmann, 2011). Is there a technology associated with PSM that can be assessed according to these principles?

Answer: Home-based technologies frequently are not tested to see if (a) they are safely and effectively usable for individuals and communities from all educational and socioeconomic status levels, (b) they are patient-centered, and (c) they have been developed with public discussion. Does their design require the patient to continue to be tethered to the provider more than is necessary?

Also, what are the technologies that have not been developed or that should be more widely available and that patients need and want? Why haven't they been developed?

5. Concern has been raised about the lack of regulation for health-related apps or smartphones, which means that the validity and reliability of their content is unknown. Apps that focus on pain relief provide education and sometimes skill training aimed at strengthening as well as tension relieving exercises and relaxation techniques. Some have opportunity for keeping a pain diary that patients must interpret (Rosser & Eccleston, 2011). What ethical concerns does this situation present?

Answer: People with pain are frequently desperate for relief and therefore especially vulnerable to being misled, yet these apps did not have quality control (Rosser & Eccleston, 2011).

6. It is said that patients' subjective experience of their illness and their sense of self are in part framed by what their technologies do for them, eliciting a sense of vulnerability without the technology. Is this arrangement manipulative?

Answer: It can be, especially if the subjectivity is directed by a marketing campaign, which frames the patient as dependent on the technology absent objective evidence of its usefulness, or if it precludes more helpful relationships/technologies. It could be positive if the technology works or is helpful in building self-efficacy or SM of the disease.

7

Paradigmatic Examples of Patient Self-Management Ethics

Policies and practices of patient self-management (PSM) and development of tools to support it often have proceeded from assumptions derived from medical practice, both its focus and philosophy, and institutional practices, particularly the payment for services system that embody these foundations. Such a restrictive framework limits the benefits that can flow outward from PSM for diagnosed illnesses and biomedical disorders; more crucially, this framework ignores the needs of persons with debilitating symptoms but no medical diagnosis or treatment plan.

SHIFTING BOUNDARIES FROM PROVIDER MANAGEMENT TO PSM (AND BACK)

Based on no particular criterion, including that of patient welfare, PSM of chronic diseases is expanding, although unevenly. We see examples of this trend in recent reports of cardiovascular and respiratory diseases, as well as other disorders that usually are diagnosed and treated by health professionals.

For some years, studies from Europe have indicated that the International normalized ratio (INR) management by self-testing can decrease hemorrhagic complications and thromboembolism by as much as 50% in patients on anticoagulants. Yet only 1% of United States warfarin patients currently self-test, and a 2005 study of U.S. anticoagulant clinics found that 60% had policies that prohibited self-testing (Wirth, 2008). At the same time, the number of dispensed prescriptions for warfarin has increased dramatically, and it has become one of the chief drugs for adverse effects (Wysocki, Nourjah, & Swartz, 2007). A recent meta-analysis found that patient self-testing (with provider-altered dosage) in conjunction with PSM (self-testing and dosage adjustment) results in significantly fewer deaths and thromboembolic events without the increased risk for a serious bleeding event; it results, too, in a better quality of life. But in half the trials fewer than 50% of potentially eligible persons successfully completed training and agreed to be randomly assigned to an intervention (Bloomfield et al., 2011). In short, PSM is not popular in the United States, yet why should patients be denied access to this approach given the encouraging findings in relevant studies?

Currently, payment for INR self-testing is withheld by Centers for Medicare and Medicaid Services until a patient has been on a stable dose of oral anticoagulant for ninety days. Yet, this is exactly the postoperative period in which rates of thromboembolism and bleeding are greatest and strict INR control by patient self-testing is most beneficial. As an illustration, Thompson, Sundt, Sarano, Santrach, and Schaff (2008) provided PSM preparation for heart valve replacement before hospital discharge and monitored patients for one month to assess both their ability to self-test and the accuracy of their INR measurements. Interestingly, in another study of self-testing, patients who returned to clinic management after the study ended carried over better control of INR in comparison with a control group. The likely reason for this outcome is that self-testing requires better patient understanding of the treatment (Ryan, O'Shea, & Byrne, 2010).

A similar pattern of ignoring research results is seen in treatment of deep venous thrombus. Between 1996 and 2006, 37 investigations showed that within constraints of appropriate patient selection and adequate outpatient infrastructure, home treatment (instead of hospitalization) would be safe and effective. But 11 years after these data became available, only a 21% decrease had occurred in population-based incidence of hospitalization among patients with this principal diagnosis (Stein, Hull, Matta, & Willyerd, 2010).

Some biomedical disorders could clearly benefit from PSM, but the approach remains underdeveloped. For example, rapid control (within 2 hours) of bleeding episodes in hemophilia minimizes joint damage and pain, improves quality of life, and reduces need for hospitalization. It is widely accepted that home treatment using bypassing agents is necessary to meet this standard. Still missing are the education and tools to help patients and caregivers recognize the bleed earlier and therefore treat earlier (Berntorp, 2011).

Documentation of the state of the science in promoting self-management (SM) in persons with heart failure exposes the gaping holes in research and in delivery of care to this large population. In this review, SM refers to decision making in response to signs and symptoms in the real world, and acknowledges that, as with other chronic diseases such as diabetes, it is impossible for a community-dwelling patient to avoid SM. Still, specific sets of SM behaviors show particular patterns of difficulties. For medication taking, studies document lack of understanding about discharge instruction as well as confusion about apparently conflicting instructions given by different physicians. Although it is common to instruct persons with heart failure to vary diuretic doses in response to changes in body weight, there is lack of clarity about adherence targets necessary for an optimal response (Riegel et al., 2009).

For symptom monitoring in heart failure, it has been demonstrated that patients delay for days before seeking care, frequently unable to recognize early symptoms as being related to heart failure. In fact, virtually every component of the health care system fails in promoting SM for persons with heart failure. While knowledge is important, patients also need skills training in how to manage their illness and when; yet, we know little about which SM skills are most problematic for these patients. Perhaps this is because skills evolve over time and practice, and most patients need assistance to master them (Riegel et al., 2009).

We see a similar picture with asthma. Although studies have shown that well-controlled asthma is achievable in the majority of patients, particularly when there is a written action plan for exacerbations, the bulk of cases treated in general practice remain uncontrolled (Chapman, Boulet, Rea, & Franssen, 2008). The rate of asthma patients in Europe with optimal control of their condition is only 5.3%, even though study findings show that introduction of PSM education increases asthma control significantly. Most persons with asthma lack awareness of the severity of their disease and the extent of airway obstruction (Kaya et al., 2009). Compounding the problem, asthmatics with severe cases of the disease (5%–10%), which are more poorly understood and difficult to control, are frequently excluded from studies of PSM preparation (Smith, Mugford, Holland, Noble, & Harrison, 2007).

On the other hand, findings point to usefulness of PSM in patients with chronic obstructive pulmonary disease, especially in recognizing stages of increasing breathlessness and in early recognition of exacerbations. Trials showed that early treatment stimulated by adherence to a written action plan (part of a PSM program) (Bischoff et al., 2011) leads to faster symptom recovery (Bourbeau, 2009).

Another trial combined pain SM with antidepressant therapy and produced substantial reduction in depression severity and remission rates and moderate reduction in pain severity and pain-related disability (Kroenke et al., 2009). And a rehabilitation program for chronic knee pain gave people a SM strategy of exercise that decreased pain and changed patient beliefs about the safety and utility of exercise to control symptoms (Hurley, Walsh, Bhavnani, Britten, & Stevenson, 2010).

Dialysis for kidney failure represents a switch from PSM (home hemodialysis), prominent in the 1960s, to the treatment being provided by professionals in centers. Currently, many dialysis programs do not have the expertise to offer home hemodialysis or peritoneal dialysis as a patient choice; such protocol is influenced by lack of adequate reimbursement for patient education about modality choice and a physician reimbursement system favoring in-center dialysis (Qamar, Bender, Rault, & Piraino, 2009). Again, such a trend seems unrelated to criteria of patient safety and preference.

The ethical concerns common to the shifting boundaries between provider- and patient-delivered care reflect the bases underlying these moves. When the shift is to patients, how can we ensure safety while promoting PSM? Equally of concern is the option for professional retention of care that should/could be provided by patients. At any rate, while other factors are likely involved, two that commonly restrain the flow of known benefits to patients who could self-manage their condition are lack of payment policies supporting provider time for initial preparation for SM and ongoing support to patients, and a reimbursement system totally focused on medical procedures. In fact, PSM as a philosophy of care is much more prominent in nursing than in medicine, especially advanced practice nursing.

CONTRIBUTION OF PSM TO DECREASE OF HEALTH DISPARITIES AND POVERTY

Ironically, the medical field has been slow to promote PSM for diseases associated with low income populations. It is reasonable to suppose that if an adequate degree and caliber of SM controls symptoms and potentially slows disease progression, individuals will be able to work and go to school, removing one element (bad health) that keeps them in poverty. For diseases common in families and communities, it is also reasonable to think that investment in good SM skills will yield benefits to other members, including across generations. However, little research addresses these potentials.

As a rare instance, intergenerational transmission of chronic illness PSM expertise has been studied in African American families with hypertension, which is particularly important because of the high prevalence and early onset of the disease in this population. Among this group, lack of knowledge and self-efficacy for medication adherence has been associated with the inability to control blood pressure. In addition, studies suggest that older parents directly influence adult children in their knowledge about PSM (Warren-Findlow, Seymour, & Shenk, 2011).

Some infectious diseases that become chronic also must be self-managed. HIV/AIDS is one well-known example. A lesser known example is hepatitis C virus (HCV), which has received some attention for PSM. This disease infects about 2% of the U.S. population and often co-occurs with substance problems, homelessness, and impoverishment. Long-term consequences include cirrhosis, hepatocellular carcinoma and need for liver transplant, and functional limitations leading to an impaired quality of life. Groessl et al. (2011) studied a Veterans Affairs population with HCV. Only about 20% of this population ever sought antiviral treatment, but the study showed that the PSM program could improve overall health and independence from antiviral therapy. This is important because there are few, if any, interventions available for HCV-infected individuals who have failed or are not immediate candidates for antiviral therapy, a subpopulation that constitutes almost 75% of HCV-infected persons (Groessl et al., 2011).

This program added condition-specific modules to Lorig's Chronic Disease Self-Management Program, which teaches problem solving, engages patients in day-to-day management of their illness and incorporates role and emotional management. Modules specific to HCV addressed substance use disorders and treatment communication with health providers through use of action plans comprised of small behavioral changes and reports to a health professional and a peer co-leader (Groessl et al., 2011).

PERSONS WITH DEBILITATING SYMPTOMS BUT WITHOUT MEDICAL DIAGNOSIS AND/OR TREATMENT PLAN

Because the diagnostic phase is frequently long and medical treatment often lacking for neurological disease, including for problematic symptoms, PSM is undeveloped in this area. Where it has been documented, the effectiveness of PSM is likely due both to patient monitoring and therapy adjustment and to nonspecific effects of coping support. These documented outcomes raise ethical questions about whether neurology patients should be denied PSM options.

As a specific example, in the aftermath of diagnosis, persons with multiple sclerosis (MS) confronting relative absence of viable management and treatment recommendations often felt they were encouraged to prepare for life as an invalid rather than active engagement in SM. In fact, health professionals may interpret active SM among such patients as a form of psychological denial (Thorne, Harris, Mahoney, Con, & McGuinness, 2004).

Fortunately, a slow accumulation of research findings about educational approaches for PSM in neurological disease is becoming available. An online fatigue management program not only provides skills but self-confidence and connection with others coping with issues common in MS (Ghahari, Packer, & Passmore, 2009). And a small study suggests these patients may need special learning approaches. This sample perceived themselves as less competent than others, at some cost to their self-esteem. When problem-solving they moved toward obvious solutions that didn't require much consideration of alternatives, and avoided emotional and cognitive complexity and a long-range view. Thus, patients with neurological chronic disease may need more guidance in considering the risks and benefits of treatment choices (Ozura, Erdberg, & Sega, 2010).

For some common conditions such as low back pain, there is no definitive treatment that provides relief. In this situation patients must learn through experimenting with exercise and medication how to interpret pain signals and manage them, deciding when to extend oneself and when to rest, gradually moving toward feeling in control. Indeed, PSM for control of chronic low back pain has yielded improved daily functioning and quality of life results comparable to spinal surgery (van Hooff et al., 2010). Alternatively, both fear of pain and beliefs that it cannot be controlled may well transition to disability (Damsgard, Dewar, Roe, & Hamran, 2011), a situation with great costs to the individual and to society.

PATIENTS WITH COMORBIDITIES

Although comorbidities are common in chronic disease, little attention has been paid to establishing guidelines for meshing PSM regimens for multiple conditions. This is probably because multiple regimens tend to conflict. What is challenging in these situations is that patients may choose which conflicting elements to abandon, with unknown safety consequences.

We find an example in individuals with schizophrenia. In this population type 2 diabetes mellitus is two to four times more prevalent than in the general population, with estimated rates of 15% to 25%. Antipsychotic medications can increase risk of developing diabetes, and schizophrenia may impair cognitive function, including the learning and motivation necessary for PSM. Although very few studies have evaluated diabetes control in this population, persons with schizophrenia and chronic mood disorders have less diabetes education and have found diabetes SM difficult when psychotic symptoms are severe. A small cross-sectional study testing this hypothesis found mixed evidence (Ogawa, Miyamoto, & Kawakami, 2011).

A further example in heart failure shows that due to comorbid conditions, as many as one-third of patients are trying to follow two different diets, with another third trying to follow three different diets. Comorbidities in heart failure also make symptom monitoring difficult; persons with comorbid lung disease may find it difficult to distinguish dyspnea that could be caused by either or both of these conditions (Riegel et al., 2009). A study in the United Kingdom found that the number of symptoms people experience is higher for persons with chronic conditions (McAteer, Elliott, & Hannaford, 2011), meaning they have a larger burden of ascertaining the significance of their symptoms and whether professional care should be sought. Typically, practice guidelines for health professionals (and patients) are single-disease focused and do not provide guidance for how comorbidities may affect the treatment plan and SM practice of patients.

This work on PSM of comorbid conditions is the very start of studies we need that include descriptions of how conflicting regimens for multiple chronic diseases have been or could be resolved by providers and patients. Indeed, Starfield (2011) has suggested that maintaining a disease-by-disease focus, as is seen in the current organization of the PSM of chronic disease literature, is counterproductive. Diseases are heterogeneous and never clearly distinct entities, and multimorbidity is not just the sum of individual disease diagnoses. Rather, it is the degree of comorbidity that influences resources (Starfield, 2011).

Primary care professionals have reported difficulties in managing patients with multimorbidities within the consultation time and have been found to deal with chronic conditions according to priority and deferring those not attended to. Providers could not describe a specific decision-making model around managing multimorbidity, even though there are clearly interactions between conditions (disease entities). The United Kingdom provides financial incentives for quality of care, but these incentives relate to single conditions. And the overall structure of the health care system, not organized for multimoribidity, requires patients to attend many individual disease clinics, yielding contested priorities. Such a situation results in low patient capacity for SM (Bower et al., 2011).

MENTAL HEALTH RECOVERY MOVEMENT

As a follow up to our discussion of comorbidities, not only is mental illness frequently a chronic disease, it also affects occurrence, treatment, and outcome of other chronic diseases. Remarkably, beginning in the late 1980s, mental health has become a laboratory for various approaches to PSM, including a full-blown social and moral movement to change the ends from chronic treatment to recovery. In some ways the movement was transformative, reworking traditional power relationships and conferring distinctive expertise on service users and their ability to negotiate treatment, with foci on (1) choice, self-direction and empowerment; (2) regaining competence; (3) and moral agency. This development was a correction to notions of inevitable decline, bearing a striking similarity to the capabilities approach outlined in Chapter 1.

Consistent with PSM in other illnesses, recovery in mental illness does not necessarily require an absence of symptoms but instead their management, thus illness and recovery can occur at the same time. The overall message is that patients may find medication helpful while learning SM skills, versus resigning to taking medication for life. For example, sufferers learn how to cope with mood swings. These are autonomy-enhancing approaches, focused on capabilities and successes, not problems and deficits (Hopper, 2007).

Although many interventions whose benefits are already scientifically established (including psychoeducation) are barely available to mental illness persons (Amering & Schmolke, 2009), it is fair to say that measurement of recovery and establishment of a strong evidence base are in development. Yet studies display little consensus for "recovery" and do not capture real-life situations (Shrivastava, Johnston, Shah, & Bureau, 2010), and little is known about their validity for predicting real world outcomes, certainly not in the long run (Mausbach, Moore, Bowie, Cardenas, & Patterson, 2009). So far we know that improvement or remission of symptoms (hallucinations and delusions) is not necessarily linked to improvement in functioning (Mausbach et al., 2009).

What the mental health recovery movement does show is that PSM is important, even necessary, for most chronic illnesses, and that development of agency and capabilities is not only ethically relevant but an inherent part of PSM.

Traditional treatment of one mental health problem, bipolar disorder, illustrates the potential divergences of a PSM approach. It can take almost a decade to establish a bipolar diagnosis. Once identified, the primary focus for mental health care has been centered on treating the illness and controlling the symptoms. Consistent with the medical approach, outcome measures have included time to relapse, length of stay in hospital, and compliance with pharmacologic treatment. Facilitating daily management of the affected person and family remains lacking. A study found it difficult for patients to distinguish between their own normal way of feeling and what was illness-related, and families felt guilty as they questioned their approach to the affected family member. Educational interventions increased PSM capability and instilled in patients an ability to influence their illness and live a manageable life (Jonsson, 2010).

Colom et al. (2009) found that a 21-session psycho-educational program aimed at PSM of bipolar disorders also resulted in fewer recurrences and less time acutely ill or hospitalized, at both the 2- and 5-year follow up. The program targeted improving illness awareness, treatment adherence, early detection of prodromal symptoms and recurrences, and lifestyle regularity. A few individuals reported transient increased anxiety and fear or ruminations related to the psycho-education. Such side effects should be monitored.

Nonetheless, it is important to note the ways in which the PSM, as developed for chronic physiological conditions such as diabetes and heart disease, doesn't fit SM of mental illnesses such as bipolar disorder. PSM assumes a true, coherent, stable, rational patient fully distinguishable from disease, one who can observe, anticipate, and preside over it. In the case of bipolar disorder, rationality of the patient is called into question, the patient may not be seen as fully rational and the disease that is managed coincides with the self. These patients must practice constant surveillance of their thoughts and emotions but often can be trained to develop a form of self-managing agency to tell the difference between the "well self" and the "self that is ill," and not be fooled (Weiner, 2011).

COMMON CHRONIC CONDITIONS FOR WHICH NO STABLE PSM MODEL EXISTS

As more effective treatments become available, certain disease entities such as cancer and AIDS turn into chronic conditions for some patients. In the United States, the nearly 12 million cancer survivors include individuals whose early-stage cancer was treated and has not recurred, those with chronic forms of cancer undergoing long-term treatment, people whose cancer is likely to recur, and those with chronic cancer-related symptoms. Even so, little research on managing cancer as a chronic illness is available, even though PSM is quite relevant in this scenario. Questions include how we can structure care of cancer as a chronic disease, how patients can be helped to manage symptoms, and how patients can learn to live with the uncertainty that cancer brings (Berlinger & Gusmano, 2011)—all elements of PSM.

A second example is atrial fibrillation (AF). Associated with stroke and cardiomyopathy, AF may occur alone or with other cardiovascular conditions. Because symptoms and episodes may be too transient to confirm by electrocardiography, clinicians sometimes minimize their significance and fail to provide support and information needed for management of recurrent symptomatic AF. Delay in diagnosis is common even though it increases risk for stroke and cardiomyopathy, and providers may suggest the condition is insignificant. And because the public knows little about it, sources of support among family and friends are probably unavailable. Controversy about the best approach for treating AF means multiple providers often have conflicting advice, and despite patient adherence to the plan, treatment failure and recurrence remain high (McCabe, Schumacher, & Barnason, 2011).

Through experimentation, some patients eventually learned how to pace activities to control symptoms of AF. A qualitative study of the patient's perspective suggests that structured PSM programs for this disorder should be developed and tested (McCabe et al., 2011). This is another example where a distressing and potentially dangerous illness that doesn't fit into traditional medical practice is dismissed, missing an opportunity for meaningful PSM.

Although chronic pain is a significant symptom in a number of chronic conditions and must be managed by patients, no stable model of PSM education and support has evolved. Yet, elements of a model are emerging. As with other chronic conditions, it has been suggested that chronic pain management must focus on functional goals most important to the patient, not pain scores. Working with the patient on balancing benefits and harms of therapy helps to establish a partnership in which blame is minimized (Nicolaidis, 2011). If opioids are used, a patient-centered assessment of problems and concerns (Prescribed Opioid Difficulties Scale) is useful. Risks from opioid therapy for chronic pain have largely been defined from the provider's perspective, typically focusing on abuse and dependency. But it is possible to assess PSM of chronic pain, to identify areas where patients want help; the scale is not a screening tool to identify problem patients. A score of 8 is considered medium and a score of 16, high (Banta-Green et al., 2010).

EXHIBIT 7.1
Prescribed Opioid Difficulties Scale

Problems scale items	Concerns scale items
1. (In the past 2 weeks) Opiate medicines have caused me to lose interest in my usual activities.[a] Strongly disagree (0) Disagree (1) Neutral (2) Agree (3) Strongly agree (4)	9. (In the past 2 weeks) I have been preoccupied with or thought constantly about use of opiate pain medicines.[b] Strongly disagree (0) Disagree (1) Neutral (2) Agree (3) Strongly agree (4)
2. (In the past 2 weeks) Opiate medicines have caused me to have trouble concentrating or remembering.[a] Strongly disagree (0) Disagree (1) Neutral (2) Agree (3) Strongly agree (4)	10. In the past year, I have felt that I could not control how much or how often I used opiate medicine.[b] Strongly disagree (0) Disagree (1) Neutral (2) Agree (3) Strongly agree (4)
3. (In the past 2 weeks) Opiate medicines have caused me to feel slowed down, sluggish, or sedated.[a] Strongly disagree (0) Disagree (1) Neutral (2) Agree (3) Strongly agree (4)	11. (In the past year) I have needed to use a higher dose of opiate pain medicine to get the same effect.[b] Strongly disagree (0) Disagree (1) Neutral (2) Agree (3) Strongly agree (4)

(continued)

EXHIBIT 7.1
Prescribed Opioid Difficulties Scale *(continued)*

Problems scale items	Concerns scale items
4. (In the past 2 weeks) Opiate pain medications have caused me to feel depressed, down, or anxious.[a] Strongly disagree (0) Disagree (1) Neutral (2) Agree (3) Strongly agree (4)	12. (In the past year) I have worried that I might be dependent on or addicted to opiate pain medicines.[b] Strongly disagree (0) Disagree (1) Neutral (2) Agree (3) Strongly agree (4)
5. (In the past 2 weeks) How often have side effects of opiate medicines interfered with your work, family, or social responsibilities? Never (0) Rarely (1) Sometimes (2) Often (3) Always or almost every day (4)	13. (In the past year) I have wanted to stop using opiate pain medicines or to cut down on the amount of opiate medicines that I use.[b] Strongly disagree (0) Disagree (1) Neutral (2) Agree (3) Strongly agree (4)
6. (In the past 2 weeks) How often did opiate medicine make it hard for you to think clearly? Never (0) Rarely (1) Sometimes (2) Often (3) Always or almost every day (4)	14. In the past year, opiate medicines have caused me to have problems with family, friends, or coworkers.[b] Strongly disagree (0) Disagree (1) Neutral (2) Agree (3) Strongly agree (4)
7. In the past year, about how many times did opiate medicines make you sleepy or less alert when you were driving, operating machinery, or doing something else where you needed to be alert? Never (0) Once or twice (1) Three or more times (4)	15. (In the past year) Family or friends have thought that I may be dependent on or addicted to opiate pain medicines.[b] Strongly disagree (0) Disagree (1) Neutral (2) Agree (3) Strongly agree (4) Asked but Not Scored
8. Considering the side effects of opiate medicines you experienced in the past month, how bothersome were those side effects? Not at all bothersome (0) A little bothersome (1) Moderately bothersome (2) Very bothersome (3) Extremely bothersome (4)	16. Over the past month, how helpful have you found opiate pain medicines in relieving your pain. Not at all helpful (0) A little helpful (1) Moderately helpful (2) Very helpful (3) Extremely helpful (4)

[a]Items marked with an asterisk are scored with agree/strongly agree and assigned a 4, and all other responses are assigned a 0 for the recoded version of the scale.

[b]Items marked with an asterisk are scored with agree/strongly agree and assigned a 4, and all other responses are assigned a 0 for the recoded version of the instrument.

Source: Adapted from Banta-Green, Von Korff, Sullivan, Meririll, Doyle, & Saunders (2010), *Clinical Journal of Pain, 26*(6), pp. 489–497. Copyright © American Academy of Pain Management. Used with permission of Lippincourt Williams & Wilkins via Copyright Clearance Center.

Also of importance is recognition that chronic illness may impair normal developmental milestones, particularly in children who may need additional interventions to be successful at PSM. Social competence (evaluation of a child's level of social functioning) was found less well developed in children with chronic conditions in a meta-analysis of 57 studies, particularly for children with neurological disorders, moderately for children with blood disorders, and not at all for those with asthma and diabetes. Presumably, visibility of the illnesses as well as emotional and behavioral symptoms may play mediating roles in levels of social competence. Social skills interventions such as social problem solving, modeling and social perception training may be especially effective (Martinez, Carter, & Legato, 2011).

SUMMARY

Boundaries between medical management and PSM are societally defined, apparently frequently based on some undisclosed physician judgment and/or on systems of payment for care, which usually do not recognize PSM. Infrequently, patient groups have forced reform; in the case of the mental health recovery movement, these involved both the goals and means of care. In an era of evidence-based medicine, how can we ignore that standards incorporating patient safety and preference in PSM have not been fully developed, much less enforced?

STUDY QUESTIONS AND ANSWERS

1. After a decade of marketing modestly effective but fairly safe drugs for MS, we now have more effective but also more risky drugs. This situation precipitated development of a SM program for MS patients' education, to empower these patients to share decisions with their health care providers, and to develop their individual approaches with the disease (Heeson, Solari, Giordano, Kasper, & Kopke, 2011). Isn't this just another example of medically driven priority setting for a disease that long should have had a PSM support program?

   Answer: Yes, but part of its impetus is to keep patients safe with riskier drugs.

2. PSM, after a diagnosis of encephalitis, shows how individuals can potentially be blamed for the situation in which they find themselves, as a consequence of poor coping. Memory problems are common as are questions about who one was, or is, or can become. Yet there is little collective history about encephalitis or the community of patients who may be interested. Contact with health professionals hasn't always given the answers people sought. Some sufferers may have been misdiagnosed with a psychiatric illness. Patients interpreted advice to "self-manage" following effects of the disease with not being taken seriously and had difficulty figuring out what was "normal" functioning (Atkin, Stapley, & Easton, 2010). How can the notion of PSM avoid these difficulties?

   Answer: PSM often assumes a definitive diagnosis. One suggestion is to co-create with the patient a language that captures his or her experience, perhaps accomplished through groups of such patients if they exist. The patient can be helped to construct a narrative of the illness journey or a compilation of several narratives of different patients.

3. Different cultural contexts have required and supported different amounts of PSM. Is this justifiable?

   Answer: Yes in one sense, no in another. Yes, because cultures will simply differ in their emphasis on patient autonomy and in the values that undergird resource distribution. No, in light of evidence that PSM education and support is necessary for better disease and quality of life outcomes and to the extent that it may be cost effective and may allow alternative use of resources.

4. Paradigmatic cases represent those for which there is no clear structure emanating from the medical model, unlike those common chronic diseases reviewed in Chapter 2. What kind of model can assist the provider in dealing with ethical issues?

   Answer: A dialog with the patient will unearth the social context in which he or she experiences the illness, identify morally problematic aspects, and negotiate the most ethically satisfactory solution, which would not have been known at the beginning of the conversation. For further exploration of this model, refer to Ohnsorge and Widdershoven (2011).

5. Shifting the boundaries between providers and patients in chronic illness care can be confusing. At least two perspectives are currently in mode: evidence-based health care and patient-centered care. Clinicians and systems of care try to integrate these visions. Patient responsibility discourses can overestimate the ability of a patient to control disease activity. Patient responsibility to comply can be described as paternalism. Evidence-based language can create a false sense of security and assume that if evidence-based practice is delivered, the outcomes are no longer under the provider's control (Thille & Russell, 2010). Are any of these positions ethically appropriate?

   Answer: No—but they do suggest reasons for confusion. As in any ethically contested issue, each of these positions reflects important values, probably taken to an extreme. The stance currently thought to be most ethically justifiable is use of scientific evidence as a tool to help plan care with patients, taking their contexts, concerns, and goals into account (Thille & Russell, 2010).

6. A large concern among medical practitioners is that patients with chronic diseases do not comply with their prescribed regimens. Are these noncompliant patients simply asserting their autonomy?

   Answer: Maybe, maybe not. Noncompliance can occur for many reasons, only some of which are autonomy based. If a patient fully understands reasons and implications and chooses not to comply, refusal may be autonomy based, unless of course the patient's beliefs and fears ignore well-established facts. It is difficult to establish what percentage of noncompliance is autonomy based.

7. Paradigm cases tend to reflect ethical tensions. Broadly, what are those tensions among the several topics covered in this chapter?

Answer: Almost all are autonomy based—boundaries between providers and patients shifting to more autonomy for the latter, patients with debilitating symptoms but no diagnosis or treatment plan still believing they should receive help in dealing with their symptoms, the example of the mental health recovery movement in which patients demanded a goal of recovery versus chronic disability, and the use of life experiences and peers as an important part of treatment plans previously controlled by professionals.

8. Up to 50% of community dwelling older adults report experiencing pain, frequently in multiple sites and from multiple chronic illnesses, that interferes with normal function. Yet, the majority of recommendations found in clinical practice guidelines are based on medium- or low-quality evidence, with an extremely limited number of pain management studies involving older adults. Just on the pharmacologic side, basic questions such as the long-term safety and effectiveness of analgesic treatments, reliable predictors of treatment response, and instruments are needed to better monitor older adults who are newly started on analgesics and have narrow risk-to-benefit ratios (Reid et al., 2011). Pain always has to be self-managed, frequently in conjunction with providers. How is it possible that a symptom creating such great suffering could be so understudied?

Answer: Perhaps the state of knowledge undergirding pain PSM and treatment is paradigmatic of the reason patient and consumer groups are using many ways to directly influence research priorities, seeking to force use of public research funds to better align with patient needs. The ethical concern involves unfair distribution of public resources.

8

Implementing an Ethically Appropriate Model for Patient Self-Management

Having viewed in preceding chapters contexts of health care that utilize varying degrees and quality of patient self-management (PSM), we can now conceive a model of the approach founded on ethical precepts described in Chapter 1. But first we must determine how PSM will appear in guaranteed practice. Even though little is known descriptively about a fully supported implementation of PSM in chronic disease, for many patients it is their only choice of care due to the nature and known treatments of their conditions. The visible research literature has in many instances verified benefits of PSM while not exploring its potential harms, and at the same time exposed extremely low availability of ongoing education and support. In both its goal definition and spotty implementation, PSM has been captured largely by the medical care system, which considers the approach optional. Noteworthy exceptions are community-based, layperson-led programs, which emphasize development of self-efficacy and management of psychosocial adjustments to chronic disease.

Drawing on insights from previous chapters, then, this chapter suggests how an ethically appropriate model for PSM might be implemented.

UNIVERSAL ACCESS TO SAFE AND EFFECTIVE PSM EDUCATION AND SUPPORT

As a health care practice driven by social policy, PSM represents an opportunity for more effective and efficient management of the huge burden of chronic disease across the world, as well as an opportunity for individuals and families to live a more autonomous and productive life. But PSM is largely a movement in which the tools, standards, and delivery system that would make it widely safe and available and allow it to reach either social policy goals or accepted moral practice remain underdeveloped. This volume contributes to their development by raising our awareness of ethical issues that up to now have been ignored. For example, the following untenable assumptions must be replaced:

1. Adherence to the rules and practices of directive medical expertise (the current system) is the safest and most satisfactory way to live with chronic disease, or at least, the most politically sustainable.

2. Individuals can learn and manage the complex clinical decisions involved in their treatment without ongoing, ready access to competent PSM support over time.

3. Cumulative development of health capabilities is no one's responsibility.

4. Investment in developing tools, standards, and capacity for PSM is desirable only if it is cost effective—a standard to which few other health care interventions are held. This is based in part on the misconception that benefits from PSM are private goods, that is, beneficial solely to the persons involved.

Each of these false assumptions can be countered with actualities. First, we know that PSM can be safer than current medical practice. In fact, an unprecedented theoretical consensus exists today that paternalism in medicine is mostly unacceptable. Even so, PSM opportunities remain largely under the nontransparent control of medicine and individual physicians, potentially denying patients the benefits that accrue from supported PSM. Second, recognizing chronically ill patients' right to learn a competent level of self-management (SM) requires moving beyond a framework that privileges medical diagnosis and an evidence base largely constructed with middle-class lifestyles and resources, ignoring the aged and those with complicated diseases and multiple morbidities. Everyone outside the framework of middle-class "normalcy" is a deficit, belonging to groups for which there are no answers. In contrast, and countering the third erroneous claim, a framework built around capabilities would focus on developing patient ability to monitor data and cohere it into complex clinical judgments, converting these findings into actions, with access to competent professional support to optimize benefits and detect and correct harms.

As for the fourth claim, descriptions of PSM education and support for building individual capacities still show evidence of confusion with educational models appropriate to schools. School education is a platform technology, a basic instrument used by all cultural institutions by which individuals and groups learn approved information. It focuses largely on mastering cognitive disciplines undergirded by basic literacy and numeracy skills. In contrast, in the health setting patient education orients to decisions and actions with high emotional content and often profound consequences, and should therefore protect and display all care options and serve individuals possessing a wide range of literacy and numeracy skills. One ethical concern about the confusion between school and health learning is that currently the latter automatically excludes persons who lack a high level of formal education. It assumes, wrongly, that patients must understand the theoretical base for a diagnosis and treatment plan to receive PSM support.

A second concern with confounding school and patient education is that the former is oriented to reproducing current culture and power relationships. In health care, a parallel goal has been to focus PSM education on compliance with the physician's regimen (a dominant power relationship) instead of teaching patients how to counter that advice with their learned experience and choose different end points for their care.

Perhaps a more basic philosophy, outlined by Faden, Beauchamp, and Kass (2011), should guide us. Learning at all levels of the health care system is morally essential, not morally optional, and grounded in the critical role learning plays in achieving and sustaining a socially just health care system. In such a system present and future generations have guaranteed access to adequate and high-quality health care services without generating undue financial burdens on patients and families. We have a responsibility to construct a tighter integration between research and practice in order to provide the knowledge base necessary for the system to become more equitable (Faden et al., 2011). Because access to education and support for PSM of chronic disease can be characterized as having been less than inclusive up to this point, concentrated efforts should be put in place to construct, by constant improvement to our present system, effective models by which all patients can learn to self-manage effectively along with the delivery systems that ensure such services.

GUARANTEED THRESHOLD OF CAPABILITIES DEVELOPMENT

As described in Chapter 1, capability theory addresses general skills, but it is useful to consider a more concrete example of this approach in order to demonstrate the deficiencies of current practice. It is estimated that among the U.S. population, 23 million individuals (15%) have chronic kidney disease (CKD), among whom probably one-fifth have limited school and health literacy. Most people with this condition are unaware they have kidney disease, yet nearly all therapies aimed at preventing CKD progression and decreasing the associated complications rely heavily on PSM. Among patients receiving peritoneal dialysis, higher kidney disease-specific knowledge is associated with lower rates of peritonitis. And educational interventions have been shown to delay initiation of dialysis therapy and decrease the risk of death. Yet, among a cohort of patients seeing nephrologists, one-third reported knowing little or nothing about their own CKD, and nearly half had no knowledge about treatment options if their kidneys failed (Wright, Wallston, Elasy, Ikizler, & Cavanaugh, 2011).

Against this background, the Medicare Improvements for Patients and Providers Act, passed in 2008 and administered through the Centers for Medicare and Medicaid Services, provides an education benefit on referral of a physician managing a kidney condition. The education sessions are required by law and provide information regarding management of comorbid conditions, measures to take to delay need for dialysis therapy, and how to prevent complications and seek options for renal replacement therapy (Young, Chan, Yevzlin, & Becker, 2011). This is taking education for PSM in the right direction, yet the need for this education (and indeed patients' rightful expectation that they should receive it) has existed for more than three decades.

Within and outside the United States, the capabilities approach can enact a sound and ethically appropriate model of PSM. In developed countries, we can ascertain that expenditures in the education system will translate into savings in the health sector as individuals gain the skills to quickly learn SM decisions and detect their inevitable chronic disease(s) when they appear. Even the undereducated in developed countries can improve their ability to collaborate with providers in management of chronic disease.

But most important to remember is that capabilities have value in and of themselves as spheres of freedom and choice, not just related to how they will function in a health care system. In that light, Nussbaum (2011) reminds us that there is a huge moral difference between a policy that promotes health and one that promotes health capabilities—the latter, not the former, honors the person's lifestyle choices. People from all walks of life need capability security; poverty can be seen as a heterogeneous failure of opportunity (Nussbaum).

In fact, the popular notion of disadvantage suggests that individuals from low socioeconomic status are a permanent underclass, and in the case of chronic disease, it would be prohibitively expensive to prepare and sustain PSM for this population. But the capabilities perspective sees disadvantage as not necessarily equal to poverty but as a lack of genuine opportunity for secure functioning, a lack that cannot be sustained over time. Several disadvantages may cluster together but can be broken by interventions such as education.

Two points are important. First, while societies have a responsibility to use resources efficiently, it has been argued that several moral claims by the least advantaged should override a pecuniary outlook. Second, aspects of the social structure are just as important in determining genuine opportunity for secure functioning as are individual internal and external resources. Yet, it seems easier to implement personal responsibility than to reform social structures (Wolff & de-Shalit, 2007).

TOOLS FOR PSM AND DECISION SUPPORT

One essential tool to improving the model of PSM in health care is gaining knowledge of the role played by cultural values. Historically, PSM support has largely targeted the health behaviors of individuals, an approach limiting its effectiveness considerably by at least two factors. First, case-by-case medical advice is based on the construct that risk is manageable because it can be predicted and therefore decreased or eliminated. But prognosis, treatments, and experience of chronic illnesses are ambiguous, and accumulated knowledge about how to be healthy within these conditions is constantly changing and often contradictory. Therefore multiple or "divergent" lifestyle practices cannot be convincingly disconfirmed by medical science as countering health prognosis; instead, lifestyles are chosen by whatever evidence people find convincing along with a combination of individual and cultural values. Furthermore, lifestyle choices are embedded in class and cultural "enclaves," with the poor often discounting as unaffordable the living standards approved by the medical community (Wasserman & Hinote, 2011).

A second and related means for improvement is gauging the influence of social networks that describe PSM of chronic illness. PSM takes place in different everyday worlds, embedded in everyday lived experience within various social networks. Such networks shape understanding of the self and normality, knowledge and narratives, locus of individual responsibility, patient experiences, and the kinds of consultations sought. Understanding different kinds of social networks, those which produce inequalities and those conducive to managing chronic disease and the interventions to achieve optimal conditions (Vassilev et al., 2011), will offer a new tool for more effective PSM.

NECESSARY HEALTH SYSTEM CHANGES

Changes to the structural system of health care are necessary for a definitive implementation of PSM. As a first reconceptualization, every society (local or national), no matter the size of its health expenditure, believes it has a resource shortage, a conviction that directs the focus of discussion on rationing instead of on producing optimal value. Wennberg's (2010) studies of small-area variations in care intensities in the United States conclude that if using organized practices, the country already has more than enough resources to care for all Americans. Yet for patients with severe chronic illness, care is primarily driven by capacity of the local delivery system rather than by the wishes of patients and their families. In the absence of evidence-based standards for physician visits or hospitalizations of the chronically ill, local service can be overused to expend the supply of resources (physicians and hospital beds), leading to potentially harmful overuse of treatment, both physically and economically. Wennberg's (2010) analysis suggests a need for several simultaneous reforms: democratization of the physician-patient relationship, efficient care coordination across multiple caregivers and settings over time, and adjustment of care resource capacity to match that of low-rate regions with good quality of care.

A question to ask is, how much chronic disease can we expect in the future? Thirty years ago the notion of compression of morbidity suggested that increased life expectancy would be accompanied by a shortening in the length of morbidity and that disease progression could be halted before disability. A summary of evidence from the intervening years suggests that compression of morbidity is illusory and that as the human life span lengthens, time in which need for treatment of disease increases as well as do its associated costs (Crimmins & Beltran-Sanchez, 2011).

As another crucial change needed, consistent evidence of the importance of PSM specialist roles such as asthma educators, diabetes educators, and other roles performed by health professionals (nurses and in some cases pharmacists) suggests these roles should be developed for all major chronic diseases. Furthermore, in response to education concerns documented in this and earlier chapters, these professionals and their organizations must be prepared to focus on setting standards linked to outcomes important to patients. These patient education outcome associations then become informal but powerful norm setters, operating transnationally and laying out blueprints for legitimate, universal action. It is only through such vigorous attention that the quality of PSM and support of it will reach the policy agenda. While organizations that accredit health care institutions have issued supportive statements, their agendas are basically captured by medicine, blocking vigorous action on PSM.

In addition to expanding specialist roles, an appropriate model of PSM considers the availability of support services, including medical personnel. For example, proper patient preparation for hospital discharge depends on adequate RN staffing hours. Patients have reported better quality discharge teaching, leading to a perception of readiness that influenced their application of post discharge education when staffing hours were higher. The need for adequate staffing hours is partly founded on concern about symptoms and complications that stem from failure to follow home instructions or from inadequate knowledge about recovery. Assessments of quality discharge teaching and discharge readiness are not standard pre-discharge practices, either for purposes of quality measurement or for correction of misunderstandings, but they should be (Weiss, Yakusheva, & Bobay, 2011).

Lastly, in collaboration with patient groups, the health care community should develop a new infusion of patient-oriented outcome measures that support practical inferences. To illustrate the lag in this area, only 20% of published diabetes trials designated their primary end points as outcomes important to patients. Yet a survey of more than 2,000 patients found that a quarter felt the traditional marker of HbA1c was of primary interest. It is important to recognize that patients with chronic conditions rate certain outcomes as more important than those currently used by researchers (Murad et al., 2011). Similarly, online programs such as *patientslikeme.com* are a personal research platform for patients to share their experiences using patient-reported outcomes. Patients learn from the aggregated data reports of others how to improve their outcomes, which may include changing their physicians (Wicks et al., 2010).

PSM OF CHRONIC DISEASE IN LOW-AND MIDDLE-INCOME COUNTRIES

In this volume the setting for PSM has occurred mainly in developed countries; still, shocking and avoidable statistics are seen in worldwide settings (see Exhibit 8.1). Myths about these illnesses may contribute to their

Exhibit 8.1
Burden of Non communicable Disease

- 36 million deaths a year, 63% of global deaths
- 80% of deaths from cardiovascular and diabetes and almost 90% of deaths from COPD occur in low- and middle-income countries.
- 29% of deaths from non communicable diseases in low- and middle-income countries occur in people under 60 compared with 13% in high income countries.
- Deaths are projected to increase by 15% between 2010 and 2020 with increases of 20% in Africa, the Middle East, and South East Asia.
- Almost 6 million people a year die from tobacco use, 3.2 million from physical inactivity, 2.3 million from the harmful use of alcohol, 7.8 million from raised blood pressure, and 2.8 million from being overweight or obese. 12.7 million new cases of cancer in 2008 will increase to 21.4 million by 2030, with two-thirds of cases being in low- and middle-income countries.
- The 12.7 million new cases of cancer in 2008 will increase to 21.4 million by 2030, with two-thirds of cases being in low- and middle-income countries.
- Non communicable disease accounted for five of the six top causes of economic loss in 2008.
- Non communicable diseases are a major cause of families falling into poverty, and they block economic development.

Source: Reproduced from "Global Response to Non-communicable Disease," by United Health, National Heart, Lung, and Blood Institute Centers of Excellence, M. T. Cerqueira, A. Cravioto, N. Dianis, H. Ghannem, N. Levitt, ... R. Smith, 2011, *British Medical Journal, 342,* d3823, with permission from BMJ Publishing Group LTD.

neglect in developing nations: first, that they are diseases of affluence, second, that chronic diseases do not cause premature death in low- and middle-income countries, and third, that no cost-effective interventions exist. The situation has attracted the attention of the United Nations, in part because of the association of chronic disease with poverty and delayed progress. A strong United Nation declaration would set specific goals for reducing the incidence and burden of chronic diseases, funding these efforts and committing to audits of the impact of such policies (Piot & Ebrahim, 2010). Although PSM surely must occur in global settings, documentation of the approach in developing countries is missing in the literature.

WHAT DOES ALL THIS HAVE TO DO WITH BIOETHICS?

Bioethics is a body of knowledge and a mode of analysis addressing questions such as how to promote health; how to respond well to human disease, disability, and death; and how to govern the practice of medicine and the social uses of biomedical technology. It came of age to address a cultural lag between the new biology and the new medicine and our repositioning of normative knowledge and guidance to govern the use of that power (Jennings, 2011). Chronic disease diagnosis and management is clearly a reflection of the new biology and the new medicine, and of great importance because of its increasing population prevalence. Still, its assumptions and commitments must be examined.

As has been described throughout this volume, the values and practices currently governing PSM of chronic disease are largely those of paternalistic medicine. Although physician dominance is now mostly unacceptable in fields of care such as end-of-life, medical management of chronic disease retains control of the following aspects of PSM: determining who will be successful and the criteria of success, requiring patient adherence to physician-prescribed monitoring and treatment protocols (even when lacking scientific evidence of the superiority of the prescribed regimen), confounding quality of medical management with quality of PSM, and denying patients access to health professionals with demonstrated expertise in helping individuals to self-manage. In addition, through honoring priorities of the health care establishment illustrated by its reimbursement system, the medical community has committed great errors of omission by failing to support patients whose conditions would benefit from inclusion of PSM, including those with diseases in which PSM is required (diabetes, asthma, heart failure, and others) and by ignoring the statistically typical situation of patients trying to manage multiple comorbidities.

The first step to addressing these errors is to acknowledge the lack of quality PSM support as both an ethical issue and a failure of health policy. Framing the issue as an unacceptable form of paternalism suggests both an urgency in addressing it and a very different resolution than what is more commonly suggested, such as locking out patients thought not to be responsible while bewailing deficiencies (such as low literacy) among the socially disadvantaged groups most likely to suffer from chronic diseases and the lifetime disadvantages that flow from them.

In general, the role of bioethics is to detect, expose, and correct confusions and ambiguities in a field susceptible to conflict (Kovacs, 2010). Surprisingly, there has not been a notable revolt among patients denied PSM support, perhaps reflecting socialization into a long dominant cultural norm of physicians as comprehensive experts in health. Instead, most of the conflict has come from nurses, whose discipline highly values development and support of patient autonomy, including that of underprivileged patients. Under the current health care system, nurses do much of the work of PSM education and support but are highly constrained by the goals and conditions of the medical model.

Confusions have swirled around key elements of PSM operationalization, such as the authority under which it operates, the social commitment to it, lay regulation of medical authority by noncompliance with it, and whether/how to develop other practices. Confusions have risen, too, when conceiving of PSM as a technical versus a social and moral issue. Addressing these perplexities is essential to generating practical solutions to PSM weakness that can work and be widely implemented. These basic questions concerning PSM are reflected in the tools (beliefs, measurement technologies) and practices of the approach, and gaps in understanding are exposed in paradigmatic cases in Chapter 5. Alternatives to current practices and tools, fueled by changing assumptions, have been suggested throughout these chapters.

Wave I of PSM scholarship made several contributions. It captured a set of constructs essential to PSM that include ability to fulfill social roles and the importance of self-efficacy (i.e., confidence in one's ability to carry out an action) as a central goal, and it acknowledged expertise of lay group leaders in community settings dissociated from the medical world. Many studies of PSM were and are scientifically rigorous, earning sufficient respect that this body of work could be adopted by policy makers. Wave II does not replace Wave I but asks a different set of questions, inquiries related to authority and responsibility. Perhaps a future Wave III will focus on building institutions that can speak for the expertise of patients and the lay expert, building on the work that patient advocacy associations are currently doing.

It is important to note that the moral and instrumental reformation that competent PSM can secure cannot be delivered without the workforce of well-educated specialist nurses devoted to this cause. As has been documented in this book, for every disease entity in which PSM is necessary or has been tried, specialist nurses have undergone preparation to address this need within the specific condition, although frequently without the full range of skills necessary for independent practice. Such skills should include those of ethical analysis, which occurs at several levels—everyday engagement with patients learning to self-manage, construction of programs to support SM as well as policies of the institutions in which they operate, and finally at the level of conceptualizing PSM as a practice and as a support service for patients.

SUMMARY

Ethics of PSM guarantee universal access to safe and effective support for patients to learn to manage their chronic illnesses. Patient learning at all levels of the health care system is morally essential, not morally optional (Faden et al., 2011); essential, too, is a guaranteed threshold of capability development. Re-conceptualizing chronic illness care, including PSM, is necessary to meet the burgeoning amount of chronic disease in all countries. Ethical analysis should detect, expose, and correct confusions and ambiguities in a field, as this book has attempted to do.

KEY ETHICAL QUESTIONS AND ANSWERS

1. Why is it important to further develop PSM of chronic disease and the professional practice that supports it?

   Answer: It is likely not possible to improve management of chronic disease without PSM. Too many chronic diseases require regular monitoring, and medical regimens cannot anticipate all the contexts in which patients will need to self-manage their condition. Current provider support and PSM practice are not of the quality level to capture all the benefits possible.

2. How much should we worry about potential harm from PSM?

   Answer: Of course, we should try to detect harms and correct them. Although the evidence base for PSM education is not super firm, educational practice in other settings has evolved with certain safeguards not widely incorporated in PSM support. These protective practices include clear goals and frequent checks on progress toward them, full engagement with the learner, training in authentic settings, acknowledging the importance of emotion and motivations, and others features. We should incorporate these safeguards in an improved model of PSM.

3. What are the moral risks of patient-provider relationships with great power disparities?

   Answer: In these situations it is too easy to view the patient as a lesser being with a lesser moral status. The literature frequently describes differences that instigate a standoff between the professional (read medical) culture and the "lay culture," but doesn't address why it's important to respect differences and merge the two cultures in a relationship. Each party should be knowledgeable enough to catch the other's mistakes, either as they are made or during implementation of PSM practice.

4. Is the decision to promote PSM preparation and support primarily based on a robust evidence base about its level of effectiveness, or is it founded on a well-reasoned ethical argument?

   Answer: It's based on both, but this author would argue that ethics is the foremost concern—patients have a moral (and frequently legal) right to information about their own health and the right to skills training in how to optimize it. Support for this norm can be found in policy statements including nursing licensure laws and codes of ethics. While use of the best available evidence is a practice obligation, evidence alone does not determine what we should do. We should remember two failings of evidence: (1) research data can be distorted by methodological failings in the design and reporting of trials, or by bias; and (2) norms and ethical theories can lead to other choices than those proposed by research findings. Thus, there is an inherent moral propensity to the prediction and dissemination of evidence—it can mislead, enhance, or diminish individuals' and communities' lives (Borry, Schotsmans, & Dierickx, 2006).

5. **What is the danger that PSM will be dismissed based on studies that don't optimize the intervention?**

Answer: Great danger. A good example can be found in a recent review article about patient ability to manage cancer pain, a common problem often undertreated. Although the reviewers found decreases in pain intensity and average pain in comparison with control groups, they also warned of the high risk of under-dosing the educational intervention. Trials that targeted knowledge, skills and attitudes for cancer pain and its management, as well as providing an educational dose of four or more hours with substantial follow up for reinforcement, were significantly more likely to have positive results than trials not using this approach (Cummings et al., 2011). The optimal potency level for PSM education and support interventions is an empirical question but one that must be answered; otherwise, in a cost-conscious environment, trials with a lesser dose appear ineffective and the intervention is subsequently abandoned.

6. **In what ways is the conceptual structure of chronic disease management unsupportive of PSM?**

Answer: One such concept is the definition of treatment burden, as distinct from illness burden, and recognizing that a disease like chronic heart failure places a great deal of work on the patient. Part of this work, in which patients must strive to achieve coherence of disparate understandings of their illness experience as well as facts about treatment, is a critical and largely unarticulated idea. The total PSM labor of a disease like heart failure involves following complicated medication regimens and lifestyle changes. Patients who perceive their management plans as more demanding are less likely to adhere to treatments (Gallacher, May, Montori, & Mair, 2011); unfortunately, the blame for noncompliance usually falls on the patients.

7. There is strong evidence of a growing disparity by education level for the probability of satisfactory health outcomes with major chronic diseases such as arthritis, diabetes, heart disease, hypertension, and lung disease. The value of education in achieving better health has increased over the last 25 years. Disease prevalence for the least educated is rising and the gap in prevalence between the least and most educated is rising over time, potentially related to earlier onset of chronic disease in the less educated and the lower ability of these patients to effectively manage the disease trajectory. Protective effects of education may appear as increased exercise, healthful diet, access to technologies like home blood glucose monitoring, and ability to adhere to beneficial but difficult drug regimens (Goldman & Smith, 2011). As a societal institution, what responsibility does health care have to address education disparities?

Answer: To the degree that in this nation, we are committed to avoiding wide disparities, the health care system must play a role. There are two important elements to this argument. In the process of PSM education and support, patients learn general literacy, numeracy, and thinking skills that generalize to other areas of life. Fundamental fairness requires that patients with low literacy are also helped to learn. This includes oral communications that reduce literacy demand by limiting medical jargon, making the information personally relevant rather than abstract, and insisting on real dialogue with patients (Roter, 2011). Second, with the current standard of care there is an obligation to safety that inevitably involves complex technological and treatment regimens for which patients must be educated to be safe.

8. One could suggest that we need an ethics of transition from our current state of SM practices and its support to a more appropriately just practice. What are the important elements of an ethics of transition?

Answer: First, we should be clear about our end goal: The capability framework is a strong choice for implementing an equitable practice of PSM. Second would be to appropriately label errors in current practice as errors and make them reportable. For example, newly labeled errors would include lack of assessment of any patient with chronic disease, lack of assessment of the patient's SM competencies, and little work toward correction of them. To illustrate, patients are commonly discharged from the hospital after acute treatment of a chronic or an unrelated disease with inadequate SM skills both for the short and long term. Such neglect should be the basis for legal action and reportable to regulatory authorities such as accrediting agencies. Obviously, training of health care personnel and removal of barriers they face to giving this care are essential.

9. Some societies (the United Kingdom, Scandinavian countries) have come to a consensus that development of capability to self-manage is central to their values about health and responsibility concerning all patients and not simply a choice on the part of providers or even a patient's preference to self-manage or not. Is this position justifiable? And does it provide direction for implementation?

   Answer: An inclusive model of capacity development can be executed if it is properly debated and resources for its success are made available to both patients and providers. Such a model absolutely provides direction for implementation as the absence of any such consensus in the United States is a significant element in underdevelopment of PSM support.

10. In Germany disease management programs for diabetes were first introduced against heavy opposition by the medical profession. By 2007 half the patients with type 2 diabetes were enrolled; still, a number of physicians refused to take part. If physicians refuse to enroll in the program, their patients have to switch to another practice to participate. Szecsenyi, Rosemann, Joos, Peters-Klimm, and Miksch (2008) showed patients perceived a change toward structured care not found in patients with arthritis who had less structured care. Should it be expected that physicians who don't participate in the disease management program provide lower quality care? Critique this implementation plan.

   Answer: The policy went forward despite physician opposition but placed some patients in jeopardy of lower quality care by allowing physicians to make decisions counter to patient well-being.

11. Is it inevitable that we will always have poor and disadvantaged people who cannot self-manage their chronic diseases?

    Answer: No. While it is true that this group is quite heterogeneous and many may have poor capability of reasoning in health care, we have chosen to spend our resources elsewhere. Societies with a stronger philosophy of egalitarianism find such failures morally problematic and do something about it. In addition, there is an assumption, as yet untested, that providing PSM preparation and support to individuals from lower socioeconomic status will be an inefficient use of resources—it may in fact save resources.

12. PSM can be thought of as a grand technology co-produced by medicine and society. Can we predict how it might evolve, citing how supportive technologies, access to professional services, and moral standards could play out?

    Answer: Technology, especially electronic, will continue to expand, as there is a market for it.

    Access to professional services will be strong in some countries with health care systems oriented to primary care, especially if nurse specialist roles for the various chronic diseases include standardized education and certification. Other countries (United States) will remain oriented to specialist medical care which attends to end-stage chronic disease.

    Moral standards for PSM essentially do not exist. If you are in a leadership role, develop them. They should fully incorporate patient safety while self-managing, patient choice, and measures that reflect the range of their concerns, and accountability by institutions that deliver care.

13. One author has characterized ethical issues in hospitals as "misframed," claiming that many are actually symptoms of occupational group conflicts in the hospital, in which moral arguments are weapons in the fight (Chambliss, 1996). Do you agree?

    Answer: No. Why does this characterization (occupational group conflicts) make these concerns any less ethical? Different views of morality are embedded in different disciplines, creating dilemmas of what is right. The real dilemma is that the values of medicine are so frequently favored without any understanding of views embedded in other disciplines.

Appendix A: Measurement Instruments

A large number of measurement instruments are used for assessment and evaluation purposes in PSM, most frequently to ensure a sufficient knowledge base and self-efficacy. Instruments specific to a particular health problem may be located in the literature. This appendix focuses on several instruments (or sets of them) that are generic across PSM of chronic disease with a particular focus on their validity. Several are basic to the philosophy of PSM (empowerment, patient activation).

MEASURING PAIN SELF-EFFICACY (MILES ET AL., 2011)

Patient self-efficacy (SE; belief that a patient can perform certain behaviors in a particular environment, including adverse situations) is strongly predictive of accomplishing particular actions and PSM as a whole, and of prognosis. As an example, management of chronic pain is highlighted here. SE in people with chronic pain include one's ability to control the pain and negative emotions that it brings, maintain everyday activities, and seek and implement advice about how to control it (Miles, Pincus, Carnes, Taylor, & Underwood, 2011). SE is measured through self-report and can be modified. Measures located by Miles and others assessed available instruments against criteria including validity, readability and comprehension, reproducibility, responsiveness, and interpretability.

Five of the thirteen located instruments were assessed against these criteria, and none satisfied all of them. In particular, information about the meaning of different score ranges, including clinical minimally important differences (the smallest difference in score that patients perceive as beneficial) was uniformly missing. This situation is not unusual and hampers ability to assist patients to learn to self-manage.

PARTNERS IN HEALTH SCALE (PIH)

DEVELOPED BY M. BATTERSBY AND OTHERS

Instrument Description, Administration and Scoring Guidelines

Development of this patient self-report scale began with the clinical observation that degree of disease did not predict support patients needed to self-manage—some with mild disease required lots of support and some with severe disease very little (Battersby, Ask, Reece, Markwick, & Collins, 2003). The result is a self-rated clinical tool for assessing SM in a range of chronic conditions for individuals and populations at one time and over time. Items in this 12-item scale are scored "0" (very good) indicating high self-management, "4" indicating satisfactory self-management, and "8" low self-management.

Psychometric Properties

PIH has been tested in nearly 300 patients. Cronbach's alpha (internal consistency reliability) has ranged between .82 and .88. Factor analysis showed four key factors: knowledge (items 1, 2, 4, 8), coping (items 10, 11, 12), adherence to treatment (items 3 and 5), and recognition and management of symptoms (items 6, 7, 9). Eighty percent of the variance was found to have been likely explained by these factors. High correlations were found between patient rated and service coordinator rated PIH scores (Petkov, Harvey, & Battersby, 2010)

Critique and Summary

PIH reflects only the patient's perception of his or her abilities on the various items. Reliability is not quite as high as it should be to make judgments about individual patients. Sensitivity of PIH to intervention has apparently not yet been established.

Partners in Health Scale Items

- Item 1: Knowledge of illness.
- Item 2: Knowledge of treatment of illness.
- Item 3: Taking medication as prescribed.
- Item 4: Sharing in decisions.
- Item 5: Arranging and attending appointments.

- Item 6: Understanding of need to check and record symptoms.
- Item 7: Checking and writing down symptoms.
- Item 8: Knowledge of what to do when symptoms get worse.
- Item 9: Doing the right things when symptoms get worse.
- Item 10: Dealing with effects of illness on physical activities.
- Item 11: Dealing with effects of illness on social life.
- Item 12: Progressing toward leading a healthy life.
  (Petcov et. al., 2010)

ASSESSMENT OF CHRONIC ILLNESS CARE SCALE

DEVELOPED BY A. BONOMI AND OTHERS

Instrument Description, Administration, and Scoring Guidelines

ACIC is a twenty-five item questionnaire that asks health care providers to rate degrees of support for each of the six elements of the Chronic Care Model (CCM) in their health care delivery system. Support for PSM is one of those elements. Each item is scored 0–11, with 11 as optimal chronic care support. Scores can be summed for each scale and for the total instrument. Scores of 3–5 represent basic support, 6–8 good support, and 9–11 full CCM implementation. The instrument has been used as a quality management tool by CCM collaboratives.

Psychometric Properties

All six subscales have been found responsive to process of care improvement interventions for diabetes and heart failure. Validity is also supported by significant association of ACIC scores with ratings by external teams of depth of CCM implantation (Patel & Parchman, 2011). The German version, tested in Switzerland, required some modifications to fit the health care system of that country. The study using GACIC found scores for implementation of SM support low, congruent with other studies finding patients got information but not skills, and health professionals with inadequate training and resistant to PSM (Steurer-Stey et al., 2010).

Critique and Summary

Items on ACIC provide little detail and few examples about what fits and doesn't fit in each domain. Some say it is difficult to interpret the meaning of the total ACIC scale (Parchman, Zeber, Romero, & Pugh, 2007).

Assessment of Chronic Illness Care, Version 3.5

Please complete the following information about you and your organization. This information will not be disclosed to anyone besides the ICIC/IHI team. We would like to get your phone number and e-mail address in the event that we need to contact you/your team in the future. Please also indicate the names of persons (e.g., team members) who complete the survey with you. Later on in the survey, you will be asked to describe the process by which you completed the survey.

Your name:	Date: _____/_____/_____ Month Day Year
Organization and address:	**Names of other persons completing the survey with you:**
	1.
	2.
	3.
Your phone number: (_____) __ __ __ **-__ __ __ __**	**Your e-mail address:**

Directions for Completing the Survey

This survey is designed to help systems and provider practices move toward the "state-of-the-art" in managing chronic illness. The results can be used to help your team identify areas for improvement. Instructions are as follows:

Answer each question from the perspective of one physical site (e.g., a practice, clinic, hospital, health plan) that supports care for chronic illness.

Please provide name and type of site (e.g., Group Health Cooperative/Plan)/
_____

Answer each question regarding how your organization is doing with respect to one disease or condition.

Please specify condition: _____

For each row, **circle the point value** that best describes the level of care that currently exists in the site and condition you chose. The rows in this form present key aspects of chronic illness care. Each aspect is divided into levels showing various stages in improving chronic illness care. The stages are represented by points that range from 0 to 11. The higher point values indicate that the actions described in that box are more fully implemented.

Sum the points in each section (e.g., total part 1 score), calculate the average score (e.g., total part 1 score / number of questions), and enter these scores in the space provided at the end of each section. Then sum all of the section scores and complete the average score for the program as a whole by dividing this by 6.

For more information about how to complete the survey, please contact:

tel. 206.287.XXXX; XXXXXX@ghc.org

Improving Chronic Illness Care
A National Program of the Robert Wood Johnson Foundation
Group Health Cooperative of Puget Sound
XXXX Minor Avenue,
XXXXX, WA XXXXX

ACIC Part 1: Organization of the Healthcare Delivery System. Chronic illness management programs can be more effective if the overall system (organization) in which care is provided is oriented and led in a manner that allows for a focus on chronic illness care.

Components	Level D	Level C	Level B	Level A
Overall Organizational Leadership in Chronic Illness Care	. . . does not exist or there is a little interest.	. . . is reflected in vision statements and business plans, but no resources are specifically earmarked to execute the work.	. . . is reflected by senior leadership and specific dedicated resources (dollars and personnel).	. . . is part of the system's long term planning strategy, receive necessary resources, and specific people are held accountable.
Score	0 1 2	3 4 5	6 7 8	9 10 11
Organizational Goals for Chronic Care	. . . do not exist or are limited to one condition.	. . . exist but are not actively reviewed.	. . . are measurable and reviewed.	. . . are measurable, reviewed routinely, and are incorporated into plans for improvement.
Score	0 1 2	3 4 5	6 7 8	9 10 11
Improvement Strategy for Chronic Illness Care	. . . is ad hoc and not organized or supported consistently.	. . . utilizes ad hoc approaches for targeted problems as they emerge.	. . . utilizes a proven improvement strategy for targeted problems.	. . . includes a proven improvement strategy and uses it proactively in meeting organizational goals.
Score	0 1 2	3 4 5	6 7 8	9 10 11

(continued)

139

ACIC Part 1: Organization of the Healthcare Delivery System. Chronic illness management programs can be more effective if the overall system (organization) in which care is provided is oriented and led in a manner that allows for a focus on chronic illness care. *(continued)*

Components	Level D		Level C		Level B			Level A		
Incentives and Regulations for Chronic Illness Care	. . . are not used to influence clinical performance goals.		. . . are used to influence utilization and costs of chronic illness care.		. . . are used to support patient care goals.			. . . are used to motivate and empower providers to support patient care goals.		
Score	0	1 2	3	4 5	6	7	8	9	10	11
Senior Leaders	. . . discourage enrollment of the chronically ill.		. . . do not make improvements to chronic illness care a priority.		. . . encourage improvement efforts in chronic care.			. . . visibly participate in improvement efforts in chronic care.		
Score	0	1 2	3	4 5	6	7	8	9	10	11
Benefits	. . . discourage patient self-management or system changes.		. . . neither encourage nor discourage patient self-management or system changes.		. . . encourage patient self-management or system changes.			. . . are specifically designed to promote better chronic illness care.		
Score	0	1 2	3	4 5	6	7	8	9	10	11

Total Health Care Organization Score _____ Average Score (Health Care Org. Score / 6) _____

ACIC Part 2: Community Linkages. Linkages between the health delivery system (or provider practice) and community resources play important roles in the management of chronic illness.

Components	Level D	Level C	Level B	Level A
Linking Patients to Outside Resources	. . . is not done systematically.	. . . is limited to a list of identified community resources in an accessible format.	. . . is accomplished through a designated staff person or resource responsible for ensuring providers and patients make maximum use of community resources.	. . . is accomplished through active coordination among the health system, community service agencies, and patients.
Score	0 1 2	3 4 5	6 7 8	9 10 11
Partnerships with Community Organizations	. . . do not exist.	. . . are being considered but have not yet been implemented.	. . . are formed to develop supportive programs and policies.	. . . are actively sought to develop formal supportive programs and policies across the entire system.
Score	0 1 2	3 4 5	6 7 8	9 10 11
Regional Health Plans	. . . do not coordinate chronic illness guidelines, measures or care resources at the practice level.	. . . would consider some degree of coordination of guidelines, measures or care resources at the practice level but have not yet implemented changes.	. . . currently coordinate guidelines, measures or care resources in one or two chronic illness areas.	. . . currently coordinate chronic illness guidelines, measures and resources at the practice level for most chronic illnesses.
Score	0 1 2	3 4 5	6 7 8	9 10 11

Total Community Linkages Score _____   Average Score (Community Linkages Score / 3) _____

ACIC Part 3: Practice Level. Several components that manifest themselves at the level of the individual provider practice (e.g. individual clinic) have been shown to improve chronic illness care. These characteristics fall into general areas of self-management support, delivery system design issues that directly affect the practice, decision support, and clinical information systems.

ACIC Part 3a: Self-Management Support. Effective self-management support can help patients and families cope with the challenges of living with and treating chronic illness and reduce complications and symptoms.

Components	Level D	Level C	Level B	Level A
Assessment and Documentation of Self-Management Needs and Activities	. . . are not done.	. . . are expected.	. . . are completed in a standardized manner.	. . . are regularly assessed and recorded in standardized form linked to a treatment plan available to practice and patients.
Score	0 1 2	3 4 5	6 7 8	9 10 11
Self-Management Support	. . . is limited to the distribution of information (pamphlets, booklets).	. . . is available by referral to self-management classes or educators.	. . . is provided by trained clinical educators who are designated to do self-management support, affiliated with each practice, and see patients on referral.	. . . is provided by clinical educators affiliated with each practice, trained in patient empowerment and problem-solving methodologies, and see most patients with chronic illness.
Score	0 1 2	3 4 5	6 7 8	9 10 11

142

Components	Level D	Level C	Level B	Level A
Addressing Concerns of Patients and Families	. . . is not consistently done.	. . . is provided for specific patients and families through referral.	. . . is encouraged, and peer support, groups, and mentoring programs are available.	. . . is an integral part of care and includes systematic assessment and routine involvement in peer support, groups or mentoring programs.
Score	0 1 2	3 4 5	6 7 8	9 10 11
Effective Behavior Change Interventions and Peer Support	. . . are not available.	. . . are limited to the distribution of pamphlets, booklets or other written information.	. . . are available only by referral to specialized centers staffed by trained personnel.	. . . are readily available and an integral part of routine care.
Score	0 1 2	3 4 5	6 7 8	9 10 11

Total Self-Management Score _____   Average Score (Self-Management Score / 4) _____

ACIC Part 3b: **Decision Support.** Effective chronic illness management programs ensure that providers have access to evidence-based information necessary to care for patients—decision support. This includes evidence-based practice guidelines or protocols, specialty consultation, provider education, and activating patients to make provider teams aware of effective therapies.

Components	Level D	Level C	Level B	Level A
Evidence-Based Guidelines	. . . are not available.	. . . are available but are not integrated into care delivery.	. . . are available and supported by provider education.	. . . are available, supported by provider education and integrated into care through reminders and other proven provider behavior change methods.
Score	0 1 2	3 4 5	6 7 8	9 10 11
Involvement of Specialists in Improving Primary Care	. . . is primarily through traditional referral.	. . . is achieved through specialist leadership to enhance the capacity of the overall system to routinely implement guidelines.	. . . includes specialist leadership and designated specialists who provide primary care team training.	. . . includes specialist leadership and specialist involvement in improving the care of primary care patients.
Score	0 1 2	3 4 5	6 7 8	9 10 11

144

Components	Level D	Level C	Level B	Level A
Provider Education for Chronic Illness Care	. . . is provided sporadically.	. . .is provided systematically through traditional methods.	. . . is provided using optimal methods (e.g. academic detailing).	. . . includes training all practice teams in chronic illness care methods such as population-based management, and self-management support.
Score	0 1 2	3 4 5	6 7 8	9 10 11
Informing Patients about Guidelines	. . . is not done.	. . .happens on request or through system publications.	. . . is done through specific patient education materials for each guideline.	. . . includes specific materials developed for patients which describe their role in achieving guideline adherence.
Score	0 1 2	3 4 5	6 7 8	9 10 11

Total Decision Support Score_____   Average Score (Decision Support Score / 4) _____

145

ACIC Part 3c: Delivery System Design. Evidence suggests that effective chronic illness management involves more than simply adding additional interventions to a current system focused on acute care. It may necessitate changes to the organization of practice that impact provision of care.

Components	Level D	Level C	Level B	Level A
Practice Team Functioning	. . . is not addressed.	. . . is addressed by assuring the availability of individuals with appropriate training in key elements of chronic illness care.	. . . is assured by regular team meetings to address guidelines, roles and accountability, and problems in chronic illness care.	. . . is assured by teams who meet regularly and have clearly defined roles including patient self-management education, proactive follow-up, and resource coordination and other skills in chronic illness care.
Score	0 1 2	3 4 5	6 7 8	9 10 11
Practice Team Leadership	. . . is not recognized locally or by the system.	. . . is assumed by the organization to reside in specific organizational roles.	. . . is assured by the appointment of a team leader but the role in chronic illness is not defined.	. . . is guaranteed by the appointment of a team leader who assures that roles and responsibilities for chronic illness care are clearly defined.
Score	0 1 2	3 4 5	6 7 8	9 10 11
Appointment System	. . . can be used to schedule acute care visits, follow-up and preventive visits.	. . . assures scheduled follow-up with chronically ill patients.	. . . are flexible and can accommodate innovations such as customized visit length or group visits.	. . . includes organization of care that facilitates the patient seeing multiple providers in a single visit.
Score	0 1 2	3 4 5	6 7 8	9 10 11

Components	Level D	Level C	Level B	Level A
Follow-up	. . . is scheduled by patients or providers in an ad hoc fashion.	. . . is scheduled by the practice in accordance with guidelines.	. . . is assured by the practice team by monitoring patient utilization.	. . . is customized to patient needs, varies in intensity and methodology (phone, in person, email) and assures guideline follow-up.
Score	0 1 2	3 4 5	6 7 8	9 10 11
Planned Visits for Chronic Illness Care	. . . are not used.	. . . are occasionally used for complicated patients.	. . . are an option for interested patients.	. . . are used for all patients and include regular assessment, preventive interventions and attention to self-management support.
Score	0 1 2	3 4 5	6 7 8	9 10 11
Continuity of Care	. . .is not a priority.	. . .depends on written communication between primary care providers and specialists, case managers or disease management companies.	. . .between primary care providers and specialists and other relevant providers is a priority but not implemented systematically.	. . .is a high priority and all chronic disease interventions include active coordination between primary care, specialists and other relevant groups.
Score	0 1 2	3 4 5	6 7 8	9 10 11

Total Delivery System Design Score_____   Average Score (Delivery System Design Score / 6)_____

ACIC Part 3d: Clinical Information Systems. Timely, useful information about individual patients and populations of patients with chronic conditions is a critical feature of effective programs, especially those that employ population-based approaches.[8]

Components	Level D	Level C	Level B	Level A
Registry (list of patients with specific conditions)	. . . is not available.	. . . includes name, diagnosis, contact information and date of last contact either on paper or in a computer database.	. . . allows queries to sort sub-populations by clinical priorities.	. . . is tied to guidelines which provide prompts and reminders about needed services.
Score	0 1 2	3 4 5	6 7 8	9 10 11
Reminders to Providers	. . . are not available.	. . . include general notification of the existence of a chronic illness, but does not describe needed services at time of encounter.	. . . includes indications of needed service for populations of patients through periodic reporting.	. . . includes specific information for the team about guideline adherence at the time of individual patient encounters.
Score	0 1 2	3 4 5	6 7 8	9 10 11
Feedback	. . . is not available or is non-specific to the team.	. . . is provided at infrequent intervals and is delivered impersonally.	. . . occurs at frequent enough intervals to monitor performance and is specific to the team's population.	. . . is timely, specific to the team, routine and personally delivered by a respected opinion leader to improve team performance.
Score	0 1 2	3 4 5	6 7 8	9 10 11

Components	Level D	Level C	Level B	Level A
Information about Relevant Subgroups of Patients Needing Services	. . . is not available.	. . . can only be obtained with special efforts or additional programming.	. . . can be obtained upon request but is not routinely available.	. . . is provided routinely to providers to help them deliver planned care.
Score	0 1 2	3 4 5	6 7 8	9 10 11
Patient Treatment Plans	. . . are not expected.	. . . are achieved through a standardized approach.	. . . are established collaboratively and include self management as well as clinical goals.	. . . are established collaborative an include self management as well as clinical management. Follow-up occurs and guides care at every point of service.
Score	0 1 2	3 4 5	6 7 8	9 10 11

Total Clinical Information System Score_____ Average Score (Clinical Information System Score / 5)_____

Integration of Chronic Care Model Components. Effective systems of care integrate and combine all elements of the Chronic Care Model; e.g., linking patients' self-management goals to information systems/registries.

Components	Little support	Basic support	Good support	Full support
Informing Patients about Guidelines	. . . is not done.	. . . happens on request or through system publications.	. . . is done through specific patient education materials for each guideline.	. . . includes specific materials developed for patients which describe their role in achieving guideline adherence.
Score	0 1 2	3 4 5	6 7 8	9 10 11
Information Systems/ Registries	. . . do not include patient self-management goals.	. . . include results of patient assessments (e.g., functional status rating; readiness to engage in self-management activities), but no goals.	. . . include results of patient assessments, as well as self-management goals that are developed using input from the practice team/provider and patient.	. . . include results of patient assessments, as well as self-management goals that are developed using input from the practice team and patient; and prompt reminders to the patient and/or provider about follow-up and periodic re-evaluation of goals.
Score	0 1 2	3 4 5	6 7 8	9 10 11

Components	Little support	Basic support	Good support	Full support
Community Programs	. . . do not provide feedback to the health care system/ clinic about patients' progress in their programs.	. . . provide sporadic feedback at joint meetings between the community and health care system about patients' progress in their programs.	. . . provide regular feed- back to the health care system/clinic using for- mal mechanisms (e.g., Internet progress report) about patients' progress.	. . . provide regular feed- back to the health care system about patients' progress that requires input from patients that is then used to modify programs to better meet the needs of patients.
Score	0 1 2	3 4 5	6 7 8	9 10 11
Organizational Planning for Chronic Illness Care	. . . does not involve a population-based approach.	. . . uses data from information sys- tems to plan care.	. . . uses data from information systems to proactively plan popula- tion-based care, includ- ing the development of self-management programs and partner- ships with community resources.	. . . uses systematic data and input from practice teams to proactively plan population-based care, including the development of self- management programs and community part- nerships, that include a built-in evaluation plan to determine success over time.
Score	0 1 2	3 4 5	6 7 8	9 10 11

(continued)

Integration of Chronic Care Model Components. Effective systems of care integrate and combine all elements of the Chronic Care Model; e.g., linking patients' self-management goals to information systems/registries. *(continued)*

Components	Little support	Basic support	Good support	Full support
Routine follow-up for appointments, patient assessments and goal planning	. . . is not ensured.	is sporadically done, usually for appointments only.	is ensured by assigning responsibilities to specific staff (e.g., nurse case manager).	is ensured by assigning responsibilities to specific staff (e.g., nurse case manager) who uses the registry and other prompts to co-ordinate with patients and the entire practice team.
	0 1 2	3 4 5	6 7 8	9 10 11
Guidelines for chronic illness care	. . . are not shared with patients.	. . . are given to patients who express a specific interest in self-management of their condition.	. . . are provided for all patients to help them develop effective self-management or behavior modification programs, and identify when they should see a provider.	. . . are reviewed by the practice team with the patient to devise a self-management or behavior modification program consistent with the guidelines that takes into account patient's goals and readiness to change.
	0 1 2	3 4 5	6 7 8	9 10 11

Total Integration Score (SUM items): _____ ➤ **Average Score (Integration Score/6)** = _____

Assessment of Chronic Illness Care, Version 3.5 (continued)

Briefly describe the process you used to fill out the form (e.g., reached consensus in a face-to-face meeting; filled out by the team leader in consultation with other team members as needed; each team member filled out a separate form and the responses were averaged).

Description:

_____

_____

_____

Scoring Summary
(bring forward scoring at end of each section to this page)

Total Organization of Health Care System Score _____

Total Community Linkages Score _____

Total Self-Management Score _____

Total Decision Support Score _____

Total Delivery System Design Score _____

Total Clinical Information System Score _____

Total Integration Score _____

Overall Total Program Score (Sum of all scores) _____

Average Program Score (Total Program /7) _____

What Does It Mean?

The ACIC is organized such that the highest "score" (an "11") on any individual item, subscale, or the overall score (an average of the six ACIC subscale scores) indicates optimal support for chronic illness. The lowest possible score on any given item or subscale is a "0," which corresponds to limited support for chronic illness care. The interpretation guidelines are as follows:

Between "0" and "2" = limited support for chronic illness care
Between "3" and "5" = basic support for chronic illness care
Between "6" and "8" = reasonably good support for chronic illness care
Between "9" and "11" = fully developed chronic illness care

It is fairly typical for teams to begin a collaborative with average scores below "5" on some (or all) areas of the ACIC. After all, if everyone was providing optimal care for chronic illness, there would be no need for a chronic illness collaborative or other quality improvement programs. It is also common for teams to initially believe they are providing better care for chronic illness than they actually are. As you progress in the collaborative, you will become more familiar with what an effective system of care involves. You may even notice your ACIC scores "declining" even though you have made improvements; this is most likely the result of your better understanding of what a good system of care looks like. Over time, as your understanding of good care increases and you continue to implement effective practice changes, you should see overall improvement on your ACIC scores.

PATIENT ASSESSMENT OF CHRONIC ILLNESS CARE (PACIC)

DEVELOPED BY R. GLASGOW AND OTHERS

Instrument Description, Administration and Scoring Guidelines

PACIC is the patient assessment version of ACIC, used to assess the degree that patients with chronic illness report they have received in the last six months, care that aligns with the Chronic Care Model (patient centered, proactive, and planned with collaborative goal setting, problem solving, and follow up support). PACIC consists of 20 items in five scales (please see definition in table). Each scale can be scored as an average of the items, and a summary average score can be derived. PACIC takes 2 to 5 minutes to complete, 7 to 8 minutes if administered by phone (Glasgow, Whiteside, et al., 2005).

Psychometric Properties

Cronbach's alpha for internal consistency showed .77 to 90 for the five scales, .93 for the full scale; test-retest reliability over a three month period was .58. PACIC scores were moderately correlated with scales of patient activation and problem solving, supporting its validity (Glasgow et al., 2005). Use of a guided care nurse intervention with multimorbid older patients showed better ACIC scores than usual care (Boyd et al., 2010). Because one study (Wallace, Carlson, Malone, Joyner, & DeWalt, 2010) found patient literacy in a sample of persons with diabetes to be the only variable contributing significantly to variation in SM support ratings, special attention should be paid to patients with low literacy (Wallace et al., 2010).

Culturally adapted German (Rosemann, Laux, Droesemeyer, Gensichen, & Szecsenyi, 2007) and Dutch (Wensing, van Lieshout, Jung, Hermsen, & Rosemann, 2008) versions have been developed and tested; their psychometric characteristics may be found in the cited publications. Two Australian studies found two instead of five factors (shared decision making and self management, and planned care, with alphas .88 to 95 (Taggart et al., 2011).

Critique and Summary

Scales of most relevance for PSM are those for problem solving and follow up; interestingly, patients were least likely to report receiving help with those elements. Several studies have shown that persons with diabetes report better scores than do those with other chronic diseases, usually reflecting more structured programs of care for diabetics (Glasgow, Whitesides, Nelson, & King, 2005; Wensing et al., 2008). But of most concern, most care for chronic disease occurs in primary care settings where quality of self-management support generally falls short of that documented to improve outcomes (Wallace et al., 2010), in part because in some countries solo medical practices do not include nurses who are most capable of delivering this care. PACIC can be used to establish baseline and results of quality improvement interventions in delivery of chronic illness care, using the CCM framework.

No publication has established magnitude of the PACIC score changes regarded as clinically significant. While higher levels of these elements of chronic care are related to better outcomes, it is unclear how frequently they must be provided to improve outcomes (Boyd et al., 2010).

PACIC Scale

Staying healthy can be difficult when you have a chronic illness. We would like to learn about the type of help with your condition you get from your health care team. This might include your regular doctor, his or her nurse, or physician's assistant who treats your diabetes. Your answers will be kept confidential and will not be shared with anyone else.

Think about health care you've received for your diabets **over the past 6 months**. (If it's been more than 6 months since you've seen your doctor or nurse, think about your most recent visit.)

Over the past 6 months, when receiving medical care for my diabets, I was:	Almost Never	Generally Not	Sometimes	Most of the Time	Almost Always
1. Asked for my ideas when we made a treament plan.	☐1	☐2	☐3	☐4	☐5
2. Given choices about treatment to think about.	☐1	☐2	☐3	☐4	☐5
3. Asked to talk about any problems with my medicines or their effects	☐1	☐2	☐3	☐4	☐5
4. Given a written list of things I should do not improve my health.	☐1	☐2	☐3	☐4	☐5
5. Satisfied that my care was well organized.	☐1	☐2	☐3	☐4	☐5
6. Shown how what I did to take care of my illness influence my condition.	☐1	☐2	☐3	☐4	☐5
7. Asked to talk about my goals in caring for my illness.	☐1	☐2	☐3	☐4	☐5

Think about health care you've received for your diabets **over the past 6 months**. (If it's been more than 6 months since you've seen your doctor or nurse, think about your most recent visit.)

Over the past 6 months, when receiving medical care for my diabets, I was:	Almost Never	Generally Not	Sometimes	Most of the Time	Almost Always
8. Helped to set specific goals to improve my eating or exercise.	☐1	☐2	☐3	☐4	☐5
9. Given a copy of my treatment plan.	☐1	☐2	☐3	☐4	☐5
10. Encouraged to go to a specific group or class to help me cope with my chornic illness.	☐1	☐2	☐3	☐4	☐5

	Almost Never	Generally Not	Sometimes	Most of the Time	Almost Always
11. Asked questions, either directly or on a survey, about my health habits.	$\square_1$	$\square_2$	$\square_3$	$\square_4$	$\square_5$
12. Sure that my doctor or nurse thought about my values and my traditions when they recommended treatments to me.	$\square_1$	$\square_2$	$\square_3$	$\square_4$	$\square_5$
13. Helped to make a treatment plan that I could do in my daily life.	$\square_1$	$\square_2$	$\square_3$	$\square_4$	$\square_5$
14. Helped to plan ahead so I could take care of my illness even in hard times.	$\square_1$	$\square_2$	$\square_3$	$\square_4$	$\square_5$
15. Asked how my chornic illness affects my life.	$\square_1$	$\square_2$	$\square_3$	$\square_4$	$\square_5$
16. Contacted after a visit to see how things were going.	$\square_1$	$\square_2$	$\square_3$	$\square_4$	$\square_5$

Think about health care you've received for your diabets <u>over the past 6 months</u>. (If it's been more than 6 months since you've seen your doctor or nurse, think about your most recent visit.)

<u>Over the past 6 months</u>, when receiving medical care for my diabets, I was:

	Almost Never	Generally Not	Sometimes	Most of the Time	Almost Always
17. Encouraged to attend programs in the community that could help me.	$\square_1$	$\square_2$	$\square_3$	$\square_4$	$\square_5$
18. Referred to a dietitian, health educator, or counselor.	$\square_1$	$\square_2$	$\square_3$	$\square_4$	$\square_5$
19. Told how my visits with other types of doctors, like the eye doctor or surgeon, helped my treatment.	$\square_1$	$\square_2$	$\square_3$	$\square_4$	$\square_5$
20. Asked how my visits with other doctors were going.	$\square_1$	$\square_2$	$\square_3$	$\square_4$	$\square_5$
21. Asked what I would like to discuss about my illness at that visit.	$\square_1$	$\square_2$	$\square_3$	$\square_4$	$\square_5$
22. Asked how my work, family, or social situation related to taking care of my illness.	$\square_1$	$\square_2$	$\square_3$	$\square_4$	$\square_5$

(Continued)

157

PACIC Scale (*Continued*)

23.	Helped to make plans for how to get support from my friends, family or community.	$\square_1$	$\square_2$	$\square_3$	$\square_4$	$\square_5$
24.	Told how important the things I do to take care of my illness (e.g., exercise) were for my health.	$\square_1$	$\square_2$	$\square_3$	$\square_4$	$\square_5$
25.	Set a goal together with my team for what I could do to manage my condition.	$\square_1$	$\square_2$	$\square_3$	$\square_4$	$\square_5$
26.	Given a book or monitoring log in which to record the progress I am making.	$\square_1$	$\square_2$	$\square_3$	$\square_4$	$\square_5$

SCORING INSTRUCTIONS

For PACIC Scoring:

PACIC Summary Score =	Average of first 20 items (do not include items 21-26)
Patient Activation =	Average of Items 1-3
Delivery System/Practice Design =	Average of Items 4-6
Goal Setting/Tailoring =	Average of Items 7-11
Problam Solving/Contextual =	Average of Items 12-15
Follow-up/Coordination =	Average of Items 16-20

For 5 *As* Scoring

5 *As* Summary Score =	Average of Items 1-4 and 6-16 (exclude Item 5 and average the rest)
Assess =	Average of Items 1, 11, 15, 20, 21
Advise =	Average of Items 4, 6, 9, 19, 24
Agree =	Average of Items 2, 3, 7, 8, 25
Assist =	Average of Items 10, 12, 13, 14, 26
Arrange =	Average of Items 16, 17, 18, 22, 23

Source: From Glasgow, Whitesides, Nelson, & King (2005), *Dabetes Care, 28*(11), pp. 2655–2661. Reproduced with permission of American Diabetes Association via Copyright Clearance Center.

PATIENT ACTIVATION MEASURE (PAM)

DEVELOPED BY J. H. HIBBARD AND OTHERS

Instrument Description, Administration, and Scoring Guidelines

PAM was developed to assess individuals' knowledge, skill, and confidence in managing their health (Hibbard, Mahoney, Stock, & Tusler, 2007). Activation occurs in stages: (a) believing an active role is important (assessed by items 1 and 2), (b) having confidence and knowledge to take action (items 3–8), (c) taking action (items 9–11), and (d) continuing health behaviors under stress (items 12, 13) (Skolasky et al., 2011).

Each person is assigned an "activation score," which can be computed from 0 (no activation) to 100 (high activation). One point is assigned for strongly disagreed, 2 for disagree, etc., and then scored using a calibration table (which requires a license).

Psychometric Properties

Content validity was established by a national expert panel and patient focus groups. Criterion validity was assessed by expert interview of respondents who showed lowest and highest PAM scores; no respondent was misclassified by the judges. Supporting construct validity, those with higher activation scores report significantly better health and have significantly lower rate of physician office visits, emergency department, and hospital visits (Hibbard, Stockard, Mahoney, & Tusler, 2004). Patients with high PAM scores were significantly more likely to perform SM behaviors and use SM services, with each increasing stage of PAM scores showing improved outcomes (Mosen et al., 2007). At .91, Cronbach's alpha measure of internal consistency (Hibbard et al., 2004) is high enough to use in making judgments about individual patients.

Summary and Critique

PAM can be used to assess individual patient progress as well as monitor whole populations or segment them to target interventions that vary by stage (Hibbard et al., 2007). The question of what interventions will improve activation is not well established.

Thirteen Item PAM With Item Calibrations

		Meas	SEM	Infit	Outfit
1.	When all is said and done, I am the person who is responsible for managing my health condition	38.6	0.4	0.99	0.97
2.	Taking an active role in my own health care is the most important factor in determining my health and ability to function.	41.1	0.4	1.01	0.93
3.	I am confident that I can take actions that will help prevent or minimize some symptoms or problems associated with my health condition.	41.5	0.4	0.93	0.85
4.	I know what each of my prescribed medications do.	42.5	0.5	1.05	1.01
5.	I am confident that I can tell when I need to go get medical care and when I can handle a health problem myself.	43.7	0.4	1.05	0.98
6.	I am confident that I can tell my health care provider concerns I have even when he or she does not ask	43.8	0.4	0.92	0.86
7.	I am confident that I can follow through on medical treatments I need to do at home.	45.3	0.4	0.94	0.87
8.	I understand the nature and causes of my health condition(s).	47.0	0.4	1.01	0.95
9.	I know the different medical treatment options available for my health condition.	49.8	0.4	0.92	0.87
10.	I have been able to maintain the lifestyle changes for my health that I have made.	50.5	0.4	1.04	1.01
11.	I know how to prevent further problems with my health condition.	51.2	0.4	0.96	0.92

		Meas	SEM	Infit	Outfit
12.	I am confident I can figure out solutions when new situations or problems arise with my health condition.	52.3	0.4	1.03	1.07
13.	I am confident that I can maintain lifestyle changes like diet and exercise even during times of stress.	53.0	0.4	1.05	1.11

Notes:

PAM: Patient Activation Measure.

Meas: The calibrated scale value of the item. This represents how much activation is required to endorse the item.

SEM: The standard error of measurement in estimation of the item difficulty. SEM is the precision of the item difficulty estimation and is shown in 0–100 units.

Infit: Infit mean square error is one of two quality control fit statistics assessing item dimensionality (the degree to which the item falls on the same single, real number line as the rest of the items). Infit is an information-weighted residual of observed responses from model expected responses and is most sensitive to item fit when the item is located near the person's scale location.

Outfit: Outfit mean square error fit statistic is most sensitive to item dimensionality when the item scale location is distant from the person's scale location.

Source: From Hibbard, Mahoney, Stock, & Tusler (2005), *Health Services Research*, 39/4(pt.1), pp. 1005–1026. Copyright © Health Research and Education Trust. Used with permission of Blackwell Publishing via Copyright Clearance Center.

Appendix B: Additional Study Questions and Answers

Question 1: Ethical standards do change over time. How can we describe this evolution for patient self-management (PSM) to the present time and project the evolution moving forward?

Answer: Clearly, the evolution (absolutely still incomplete) has run from expected patient compliance with a medical regimen, now to patient negotiated goals and treatment plan. Still to be resolved are patient level of responsibility in practicing the healthy behaviors thought to affect chronic disease, the negotiated treatment regimen, provider responsibility to support PSM and the unanswered question of what level of disease management and symptom control is possible in this patient.

Each of the chapters in this book raises unanswered ethical questions still accompanying this evolution; for example, potential harms of inadequate provider performance in educating patients for and supporting PSM and avoiding patient errors in practicing it, often unrecognized changes in self-identity, and ways in which measurement can entirely distort fundamental questions.

Most societies are in very early stages of addressing patient rights to PSM and responsibilities of institutions to support these rights.

Question 2: The implicit assumption of evidence based medicine is that a field like PSM needs more empirical evidence of its effectiveness, in order to be accepted by the medical profession and the public as a valid practice. What other perspectives are equally as important?

Answer: Religious, political and cultural views of chronic disease, individual responsibility for health, and the recognition of which of these important perspectives medicine currently ignores.

Question 3: How are shared decision making and informed consent alike and different from PSM of chronic disease?

Answer: All three concepts are about giving patients more authority in the patient-provider relationship. But shared decision making and informed consent occur at a moment in time, while PSM of chronic disease involves change in authority over years, often decades, in a complex relationship that involves such personal issues as lifestyle and identity, and is currently without clear guidelines about how far each party's (patient's and provider's) authority should extend.

Question 4: How do we judge if the move in health policy toward PSM is the right one—so far only a few countries like the United Kingdom have gone this direction? Is this really progress?

Answer: We are judging the policy move to support PSM on three grounds: what is the empirical evidence that it is safe and effective, does PSM save cost over the alternative, and is it congruent with patient rights/accepted notions of patient authority. While evidence for the first two is still being gathered, there is a gathering cultural shift toward more patient freedom within the relationship with providers. This last ground reflects new ethical and social norms and may be the most persuasive of all.

Question 5: Discourses of patient empowerment and development of patient agency and autonomy can conceal a real agenda of controlling costs of health care. How can such a stance be justified?

Answer: This stance can be justified by recognizing that both goals (developing patient agency and autonomy, and controlling health care costs) could be met at once. Making a concerted effort at seeing if this is possible will involve providers and patients sharing both goals and negotiating to meet them and acting on the notion that providers (as much as patients) need to be educated about PSM in the real world.

Question 6: Greenop and others note that the PSM literature on cystic fibrosis in adults is overwhelmingly concerned with patient compliance, patient deficits, and use of moral language that depicts patients as wicked, foolish, or naughty children if they don't comply with professional expectations. The frame is that patients not doing their treatments can lead only to failures. According to this analysis, the rhetoric in research and practice with these patients tries to dominate them, which can be a distinct harm to the patient, labeling the patient as morally incompetent. What alternative frame is morally acceptable?

Answer: A pragmatic, realistic, negotiated approach that recognizes limitations of known treatments and patient burden in carrying them out, realistic goals of the patient, and acknowledgment that there may not be a perfect resolution to managing cystic fibrosis. This disease, and many others, requires PSM within a largely heavily flawed medical regimen. Don't blame the patient (Greenop, Daz, Glenn, Sheila, Ledson, Martin, Walshaw, & Martin, 2010).

Question 7: How can the practice of PSM education and support keep from overemphasizing patient autonomy and independence, which, of course, are not the only important values?

Answer: By acknowledging that autonomy and independence fluctuate and that it is okay to need care from others. Many chronic diseases have nursing and medical treatments variously successful in alleviating symptoms and slowing progression. And while using these treatments and learning to give them to oneself safely requires the help of professionals, peers, and family, the patient will feel both autonomy and support from others. Benner calls this practice mutuality, leading to empowerment and growth (Benner, 2011).

Question 8: On the face of it, it seems ridiculous that patients with chronic diseases that require SM don't have a legal right to proper education and support so as to avoid harm and maximize benefit. Yet, in all developed countries, including those whose policies endorse PSM, supporting it is done poorly. How can this be?

Answer: Because such support is not yet thought of as a right. This state of affairs is diagnostic that "patient-centered care" is pure rhetoric.

Appendix C: What Can We Do?

It is important to learn from what we are discovering are our failures. This appendix documents such gaps in our practice/knowledge. How common are these problems and what can we do about them? Original sources are cited so you can read them in their entirety.

We begin with a clear message from a patient.

> What did I learn (from my experience)? Far from being lazy, most people with type 2 diabetes work hard to stay healthy. And they do so in spite of a health care system that often fails to diagnose them promptly, to teach them how to take care of themselves, and to use fully what medical science has learned about the best way to treat this disease. The system doesn't work, and yet the general attitude is to blame and punish people with diabetes—not to lend them a helping hand.

> What if we could change all that? And what if we could make it easier—even just a little bit easier for people with diabetes to do the hard work of coping with their condition?

> Our health care system clearly isn't working. It is more willing to pay for someone with diabetes to have a leg amputated than for the education, treatment and support that would have prevented the loss of the limb. (And don't even get me started on "preexisting conditions....") (Sklaroff, 2012, p. 237).

RHEUMATOID ARTHRITIS AND USE OF LANGUAGE

Fourteen focus groups across five countries and a total of 67 patients with rheumatoid arthritis (RA) provided interesting findings. Patients use the tern "flare" for multiple events; there is not standardized definition of RA flare. Patients used the word flare as a single symptomatic joint, increased symptoms within normal variation, increased symptoms from external causes such as stress or flare from overexertion. For these symptoms, patients increase their usual level of self-management by resting, pacing, applying heat or cold and escalating medications, often without seeking medical advice.

But the term "flare" can also be used to describe unprovoked, increased symptoms that are unmanageable, persistent and lead to seeking help. These complex clusterings of intense unprovoked symptoms that defy self-management are not necessarily captured in joint counts or global visual analog scales. Some patients report an early warning prodome such as flu-like feelings, fatigue or pain, sometimes appreciated only by hindsight (Hewlett et al., 2012).

BURDEN OF TREATMENT FOR PATIENTS WITH TYPE 2 DIABETES

Persons with diabetes may experience high burden of treatment and self-care demands. This study observed real primary care visits. It found that burden of treatment discussions usually arose during visits with physicians but rarely precipitated problem-solving efforts. This suggests that patients' concerns about day-to-day self-care demands were relatively unaddressed (Bohlen, Scoville, Shippee, May, & Montori, 2012).

At the time of the study no validated burden of treatment tools existed (Bohlen et al., 2012).

CHRONIC CONDITIONS AND GENDER INEQUALITIES

Women suffer more often from a wide range of chronic conditions than do men. Musculoskeletal and other pain disorders as well as mental health, account for most of the excess of poor health of women. In spite of the existence of effective for their management in primary care, these disorders have largely been overlooked in favor of other chronic diseases or cardiovascular risk factors (Malmusi, Artazcoz, Benach, & Borrell, 2011).

Gender inequalities are rooted in large inequalities in socialization, power and exposure to determinants such as employment status, income and burden of unpaid work. A health care system responsive to gender inequalities should increase its efforts in addressing the resolving this group of disorders, which have a strong impact on everyday health and well-being. Policies should include prioritization of health problems according to their impact on gender inequalities (Malmusi et al., 2011).

What might such a policy look like?

OPIOID-TAKING SKILLS AMONG PERSONS WITH CHRONIC PAIN

Patients are playing an increasingly important role in self-management of cancer related symptoms such as pain. In those with chronic cancer pain and/or those requiring opioid medication, the consequences of inadequate or inappropriate taking of these drugs can be significant (Liang, Yates, Edwards, & Tsay, 2012).

People with strong self-efficacy expectations are more likely to persist with difficult tasks even after experiencing an initial barrier or failure. Recent studies have supported this theory, showing patients who report high levels of self-efficacy re pain also report less psychological distress and physical disability (Liang et al., 2012).

The Opioid-Taking Self-Efficacy Scale—A journal for clinicians (CA) showed patients confident about some parts of managing opioid-taking but not confident about tailoring medication regimens, acquiring health and managing treatment-related concerns, especially among those with lower levels of education. Items, "change amount of pain medications if the pain returns too quickly" and "change amount of pain medications if the pain comes on suddenly," showed some of the lowest scores (Liang et al., 2012).

This is the first study to focus on assessing cancer patients' perceptions of self-efficacy in opioid analgesic taking (Liang et al., 2012).

What would you do with such findings?

ADHERENCE TO CHRONIC OBSTRUCTIVE PULMONARY DISEASE GUIDELINES AMONG PRIMARY CARE PROVIDERS

To standardize treatment for chronic obstructive pulmonary disease (COPD), an international group of experts working with the World Health Organization and the National Heart, Lung and Blood Institute (part of the National Institutes of Health) developed the Global Initiative for Chronic Obstructive Lund Disease in 1997. The main purpose of this organization was to create guidelines that would establish a standard of care for evidence-based treatment of patients with COPD (Perez, Wisnivesky, Lurslurchachai, Kleinman, & Kronish, 2012).

Subsequent studies suggest the adoption of these guidelines has been suboptimal. In this study (Perez et al., 2012), guideline adherence among primary care providers was less than 60% to five of the seven recommendations.

Adherence to the recommendation for pulmonary rehabilitation was particularly low (5%), even though this intervention has consistently been shown to decrease dyspnea and improve quality of life in persons with COPD (Perez et al., 2012).

What are the implications of such findings for patient self-management (PSM) of COPD?

PSYCHOSOCIAL BURDEN OF LIVING WITH DIABETES

Due-Christensen and others have shown that persons with type 1 diabetes benefited from support groups; major benefits were feeling less along and being intuitively understood among peers, which helped them set goals. Measured by the Problem Areas in Diabetes Scale, individuals showed significant increase in well-being although no change in HbA1C (Due-Christensen, Zoffman, Hommel, & Lau, 2012).

Psychosocial interventions usually include only patients with poor glycemic control, but in this study patients with good glycemic control had a slightly lower level of distress in living with the illness than did those with poor glycemic control but still significantly high (Due-Christensen et al., 2012). Fear of hypoglycemia and of late complications are part of distress.

At the authors' diabetes center systematic screening for patient psychosocial distress was not routinely done. It is an ethical principle that if screening is done, appropriate interventions must be available (Due-Christensen et al., 2012).

The average duration of diabetes in this study population was 21 years. The findings suggest that monitoring of diabetes distress and relevant interventions must be ongoing (Due-Christensen et al., 2012).

It should also be noted that insulin action is not always predictable, leading patients to blame themselves for being unable to control their blood glucose. The almost exclusive focus of studies in persons with type 1 diabetes has been on physical endpoints and far less on patient ability to gain mastery over their emotions related to their life with diabetes (Cradock & Cranston, 2012).

IF SELF-MONITORING OF ORAL ANTICOAGULATION IS SAFE, WHY DON'T PATIENTS HAVE ACCESS TO IT?

This summary of the evidence on this topic concludes showed a significant reduction in thromboembolic events in the group self-monitoring its anticoagulation but not for major hemorrhagic events or for death. Mean time in the therapeutic range is better in the self-management group. This analysis showed that self-monitoring and self-management of oral coagulation is a safe option for suitable patients of all ages and recommends that patients be offered the option to self-manage their disease with suitable health-care support as backup (Heneghan, Ward, Perera, & the Self-Monitoring Trialist Collaboration, 2012).

The number of patients receiving oral anticoagulants has consistently increased. Devices are available for the patient to self-test in the home setting; test results can then be managed by the health provider or patients can interpret the results and adjust their own dose of anticoagulant (self-management). Despite good effectiveness evidence, adoption of this practice has remained inconsistent in and between countries. In Germany 20% of patients on anticoagulation do self-management; in the United States this number is 1% (Heneghan et al., 2012).

Why should this situation be tolerated if capable patients want to self-manage?

WHAT ARE THE ETHICAL ISSUES IN PSM OF CHRONIC DISEASE?

Ethical analysis of the field of PSM of chronic disease has been slow to develop, either in clinical fields or in the bioethics literature. This article by Redman (2007) elaborates four issues:

- ... insufficient patient/family access to preparation that will optimize their competence to SM without harm to themselves and that will optimize benefits,
- lack of acknowledge that an ethos of patient empowerment can mask transfer of responsibility beyond patient/family competence to handle that responsibility,

- prevailing assumptions that preparation for SM cannot result in harm and that its main purpose is to deliver physician instructions,
- lack of standards for patient selection, which has the potential to exclude individuals who could benefit from learning to SM (p. 243).

Are these the most prominent issues? What others come to mind? Why have we not addressed ethical issues in this field?

IS THE DISEASE FOCUS TO MANAGING CHRONIC DISEASE AND THEIR SELF-MANAGEMENT, THE BEST APPROACH?

Chronic kidney disease is one of the comorbidities common with other chronic diseases. Some (Bowling & O'Hare, 2012) are questioning whether a disease-oriented approach is the best, especially for older individuals. Likewise, PSM has been heavily oriented to helping patients understand what is known about a disease and how to manage it.

Disease-oriented models of care assume a direct causal association between observed signs and symptoms and underlying disease pathophysiologic processes. Treatment plans target these underlying disease mechanisms with the goal of improving disease-related outcomes, an approach that may be limited especially in geriatric populations (Bowling & O'Hare, 2012).

Signs and symptoms may not reflect a single underlying pathophysiologic process. And in these populations information about safety and efficacy of treatments is often lacking because research studies have not included them. Page 296 "Coexistence of multiple chronic conditions often results in atypical clinical presentations, poor diagnostic accuracy of laboratory tests and conflicting treatment priorities. For example, pain medications for arthritis can be nephrotoxic and promote loss of kidney function" (Bowling & O'Hare, 2012, P. 296).

If a disease-oriented model has limitations, what is a better model?

Appendix D: Important Ethics Definitions

Authenticity significant emotionally appropriate living

Autonomy capacity for self-government

Communitarianism model of political organization that stresses ties of affection, kinship and a sense of common purpose and traditions

Consequentialism the view that the value of an action derives entirely from the value of its consequences

Egalitarianism a view that moral and political life should be aimed at respecting and advancing the equity of persons

Ethics the study of good, right, duty, obligation, virtue, freedom, rationality, choice

Feminism an approach to social life, philosophy and ethics that commits itself to correcting biases leading to subordination of women or disparagement of their particular experience

Libertarianism advocates the maximization of individual rights and minimization of the role of state

Deontological ethics ethics based on a notion of duty

Bioethics the branch of ethics that investigates problems arising from medical and biological practice

Measurement quantification of a thing being measured, then a rule assigning numerical values to them

Moral dilemmas situations in which each possible course of action breaches some moral binding principle

Source: From Blackburn, S., (1994). Oxford Dictionary of Philosophy, Oxford University Press.

References

Agledahl, K., Gulbrandsen, P., Forde, R., & Wifstad, A. (2011). Courteous but not curious: How doctors' politeness masks their existential neglect. A qualitative study of video-recorded patient consultations. *Journal of Medical Ethics, 37*, 650–654.

Aiken, L., Sloane, D. M., Clarke, S., Poghosyan, L., Cho, E., You, L., ... Aungsuroch, Y. (2011). Importance of work environments on hospital outcomes in nine countries. *International Journal for Quality in Health Care, 23*, 357–364.

Albano, M. G., Crozet, C., & d'Ivernois, J. F. (2008). Analysis of the 2004–2007 literature on therapeutic patient education in diabetes: Results and trends. *Acta Diabetologica, 45*, 211–219.

Alexander, J. M. (2010). Ending the liberal hegemony: Republican freedom and Amartya Sen's theory of capabilities. *Contemporary Political Theory, 9*, 5–24.

Allen, M. (2011). Is liberty bad for your health? Towards a moderate view of the robust coequality of liberty and health. *Public Health Ethics, 4*, 260–268.

Amering, M., & Schmolke, M. (2009). *Recovery in mental health: Reshaping scientific and clinical responsibilities.* New York, NY: Wiley-Blackwell.

Anderson, R. M., & Funnell, M. M. (2010). Patient empowerment: Myths and misconceptions. *Patient Education and Counseling, 79*, 277–282.

Anker, S. D., Koehler, F., & Abraham, W. T. (2011). Telemedicine and remote management of patients with heart failure. *Lancet, 378*, 731–739.

Archer, N., Fevrier-Thomas, U., Lokker, C., McKibbon, K. A., & Straus, S. E. (2011). Personal health records: A scoping review. *Journal of American Medical Informatics Association, 18*, 515–522.

Atkin, K., Stapley, S., & Easton, A. (2010). No one listens to me, nobody believes me: Self-management and the experience of living with encephalitis. *Social Science & Medicine, 71*, 386–393.

Baker, D. W., Dewalt, D. A., Schillinger, D., Hawk V, Ruo, B., Bibbins-Domingo, K., … Pignone, M. (2011). The effect of progressive, reinforcing telephone education and counseling versus brief educational intervention on knowledge, self-care behaviors and heart failure symptoms. *Journal of Cardiac Failure, 17*, 789–796.

Bandura, A. (2006). Toward a psychology of human agency. *Perspectives on Psychological Science, 1*, 168–180.

Bandura, A. (2007). Self-efficacy in health functioning. In S. Ayers, A. Baum, C. McManus, S. Newman, K. Wallston, J. Weinman, & R. West (Eds.), *Cambridge handbook of psychology, health and medicine* (2nd ed.). Cambridge, UK: Cambridge University Press.

Banta-Green, C. J., Von Korff, M., Sullivan, M. D., Merrill, J. O., Doyle, S. R., & Saunders, K. (2010). The Prescribed Opiods Difficulties Scale: A patient-centered assessment of problems and concerns. *The Clinical Journal of Pain, 26*, 489–497.

Barker, K. K., & Galardi, T. R. (2011). Dead by 50: Lay expertise and breast cancer screening. *Social Science & Medicine, 72*, 1351–1358.

Barlow, J., Wright, C., Sheasby, J., Turner, A., & Hainsworth, J. (2002). Self-management approaches for people with chronic conditions: A review. *Patient Education and Counseling, 48*, 177–187.

Battersby, M., Ask, A., Reece, M. M., Markwick, M. J., & Collins, J. P. (2003). The partners in health scale: The development and psychometric properties of a generic assessment scale for chronic condition self-management. *Australian Journal of Primary Care, 9*(2–3), 41–52.

Beauchamp, T. L. (2010). *Standing on principles.* New York, NY: Oxford University Press.

Beauchamp, T. L. (2011). Informed consent: Its history, meaning and present challenges. *Cambridge Quarterly of Healthcare Ethics, 20*, 515–523.

Benner, P. (2011). Formation in professional education: An examination of the relationship between theories of meaning and theories of self, *Journal of Medicine and Philosophy, 36*:342–353.

Berlinger, N., & Gusmano, M. (2011). Cancer chronicity: New research and policy challenges. *Journal of Health Services Research & Policy, 16*, 121–123.

Berntorp, E. (2011). Importance of rapid bleeding control in haemophilia complicated by inhibitors. *Haemophilia, 17*, 11–16.

Bischoff, E. W., Hamd, D. H., Sedeno, M., Benedetti, A., Schermer, T. R., Bernard, S., … Bourbeau, J. (2011). Effects of written action plan adherence in COPD exacerbation recovery. *Thorax, 66*, 26–31.

Bitterman, N. (2011). Design of medical devices—A home perspective. *European Journal of Internal Medicine, 22*, 39–42.

Bloomfield, H. E., Krause, A., Greer, N., Taylor, B. C., MacDonald, R., Rutks, I., ... Wilt, T. J. (2011). Meta-analysis: Effect of patient self-testing and self-management of long-term anticoagulation on major clinical outcomes. *Annals of Internal Medicine, 154*, 472–482.

Bluhm, R. (2009). Evidence-based medicine and patient autonomy. *International Journal of Feminist Approaches Bioethics, 2*(2), 134–151.

Bohlen, K., Scoville, E., Shippee, N. D., May, C. R., & Montori, V. M. (2012). Overwhelmed patients. *Diabetes Care, 35*, 47–49.

Bok, H., Mathews, D. J. H., & Rabins, P. V. (2009). Common threads. In D. J. H. Mathews, H. Bok, & P. V. Rabins (Eds.), *Personal identity and fractured selves*. Baltimore, MD: Johns Hopkins University Press.

Bonomi, A. E., Wagner, E. H., Glasgow, R. E., & VonKorff, M. (2002). Assessment of chronic illness care (ACIC): A practical tool to measure quality improvement. *Health Services Research, 37*(3), 791–820.

Boren, S. A., Wakefield, B. J., Gunlock, T. L., & Wakefield, D. S. (2009). Heart failure self-management education: A systematic review of the evidence. *International Journal of Evidence-Based Healthcare, 7*, 159–168.

Borry, P., Schotsmans, P., & Dierickx, K. (2006). Evidence-based medicine and its role in ethical decision-making. *Journal of Evaluation in Clinical Practice, 12*, 306–311.

Bourbeau, J. (2009). The role of collaborative self-management in pulmonary rehabilitation. *Seminars in Respiratory and Critical Care Medicine, 30*, 700–707.

Bower, P., Macdonald, W., Harkness, E., Gask, L., Kendrick, T., Valderas, J. M., ... Sibbald, B. (2011). Multimorbidity, service organization and clinical decision making in primary care: A qualitative study. *Family Practice, 28*, 579–587.

Bowling, C. B., & O'Hare, A. M. (2012). Managing older adults with CKD: Individualized versus disease-based approaches. *American Journal of Kidney Disease, 59*, 293–302.

Boyd, C. M., Reider, L., Frey, K., Scharfstein, D., Leff, B., Wolff, J., ... Boult, C. (2010). The effects of guided care on the perceived quality of health care for multi-morbid older persons: 18-month outcomes from a cluster-randomized controlled trial. *Journal of General Internal Medicine, 25*(3), 235–242.

Browne, T. (2011). The relationship between social networks and pathways to kidney transplant parity: evidence from black Americans in Chicago. *Social Science & Medicine, 73*, 663–667.

Brunton, S., Gough, S., Hicks, D., Weng, J., Moghissi, E., Peyrot, M., ... Barnett, A. H. (2011). A look into the future: Improving diabetes care by 2015. *Current Medical Research and Opinion, 27*(Suppl. 3), 65–72.

Bruzzese, J., Evans, D., & Kattan, M. (2009). School-based asthma programs. *Journal of Allergy and Clinical Immunology, 124*, 195–200.

Buchanan, A. (2007). Institutions, beliefs and ethics: Eugenics as a case study. *Journal of Political Philosophy, 15*, 22–45.

Buchanan, A., Cole, T., & Keohane, R. O. (2011). Justice in the diffusion of innovation. *Journal of Political Philosophy, 19*, 306–332.

Burls, A., Caron, L., Cleret de Langavant, G., Dondorp, W., Harstall, C., Pathak-Sen, E., & Hofmann, B. (2011). Tackling ethical issues in health technology assessment: A proposed framework. *International Journal of Technology Assessment Health Care, 27*, 230–237.

Bussey, H. I. (2011). Transforming oral anticoagulation by combining international normalized ratio (INR) self-testing and online automated management. *Journal of Thrombosis and Thrombolysis, 31*, 265–274

Callan, E., & Arena, D. (2009). Indoctrination. In H. Siegel (Ed.), *The Oxford handbook of philosophy of education*. New York, NY: Oxford University Press.

Carlsen, H., Dreborg, K. H., Godman, M., Hansson, S. O., Johansson, L., & Wikman-Svahn, P. (2010). Assessing socially disruptive technological change. *Technology in Society, 32*, 209–218.

Cases, A., Dempster, M., Davies, M., & Gamble, G. (2011). The experience of individuals with renal failure participating in home haemodialysis: An interpretive phenomenological analysis. *Journal of Health Psychology, 16*, 884–894.

Chambliss, D. F. (1996). *Beyond caring: Hospitals, nurses and the social organization of ethics*. Chicago, IL: University of Chicago Press.

Chapman, K. R., Boulet, L. P., Rea, R. M., & Franssen, E. (2008). Suboptimal asthma control: Prevalence, detection and consequences in general practice. *The European Respiratory Journal, 31*, 320–325.

Charlesworth, H. (2000). Martha Nussbaum's feminist internationalism. *Ethics, 111*, 64–78.

Ciemins, E., Coon, P., & Sorli, C. (2010). An analysis of data management tools for diabetes self-management: Can smart phone technology keep up? *Journal of Diabetes Science and Technology, 4*, 958–960.

Clarke, J. (2005). New labour's citizens: Activated, empowered, responsibilized, abandoned? *Critical Social Policy, 25,* 447–463.

Coleman, K., Austin, B. T., Brach, C., Wagner, E. H. (2009). Evidence on the Chronic Care Model in the new millennium. *Health Affairs (Millwood), 28,* 75–85.

Collin, R., & Apple, M. W. (2010). New literacies and new rebellions in the global age. In M. W. Apple (Ed.), *Global crises, social justice and education.* New York, NY: Routledge.

Colom, F., Vieta, E., Sanchez-Moreno, J., Palomino-Otiniano, R., Reinares, M., Goikolea, J. M., ... Martínez-Arán, A. (2009) Group psychoeducation for stabilised bipolar disorders: 5-year outcome of a randomised clinical trial. *The British Journal of Psychiatry, 194,* 260–265.

Coster, S., & Norman, I. (2009). Cochrane reviews of educational and self-management interventions to guide nursing practice: a review. *International Journal of Nursing Studies, 46,* 508–528.

Cradock, S., & Cranston, I. C. (2012). Type 1 diabetes education and care: Time for a rethink? *Diabetic Medicine, 29,* 159–160.

Crimmins, E. M., & Beltran-Sanchez, H. (2011). Mortality and morbidity trends: is there compression of morbidity? *The Journals of Gerontology. Series B, Psychological Sciences and Social Sciences, 66B,* 75–86.

Cummings, G. G., Olivo, S. A., Biondo, P. D., Stiles, C. R., Yurtseven, O., Fainsinger, R. L., & Hagen, N. A. (2011). Effectiveness of knowledge translation interventions to improve cancer pain management. *Journal of Pain and Symptom Management, 41,* 915–939.

Cutler, D. M., & Lleras-Muney, A. (2010). Understanding differences in health behaviors by education. *Journal of Health Economics, 29,* 1–28.

Dalton, A. R. H, Alshamsan, R., Majeed, A., & Millett, C. (2011). Exclusion of patients from quality measurement of diabetes care in the UK pay-for-performance programme. *Diabetic Medicine, 28,* 525–531.

Damsgard, E., Dewar, A., Roe, C., & Hamran, T. (2011). Staying active despite pain: Pain beliefs and experiences with activity-related pain in patients with chronic musculoskeletal pain. *Scandinavian Journal of Caring Sciences, 25,* 108–116.

Daniels, N. (2008). *Just health.* Cambridge, UK: University Press.

deBrantes, F., Rastogi, A., & Painter, M. (2010). Reducing potentially available complications in patients with chronic diseases: The Prometheus payment approach. *Health Services Research, 45,* 1854–1871.

Desai, A. S. & Stevenson, L. W. (2010). Connecting the circle from home to heart-failure disease management. *New England Journal of Medicine, 363*, 2364–2367.

De Vreese, L. (2011). Evidence-based medicine and progress in the medical sciences. *Journal of Evaluation in Clinical Practice, 17*, 852–856.

Dickson, V. V., & Riegel, B. (2009). Are we teaching what patients need to know? Building skills in heart failure self-care. *Heart & Lung, 38*, 253–261.

Dilorio, C., Bamps, Y., Walker, E. R., & Escoffery, C. (2011). Results of a research study evaluating WebEase, an online epilepsy self-management program. *Epilepsy & Behavior, 22*, 469–474.

Due-Christensen, M., Zoffman, V., Hommel, E., & Lau, M. (2012). Can sharing experiences in groups reduce the burden of living with diabetes, regardless of glycaemic control? *Diabetic Medicine, 29*, 251–256.

Earnshaw, V. A., & Quinn, D. M. (in press). The impact of stigma in health care on people living with chronic illnesses. *Journal of Health Psychology.*

Ebeling, M. (2011). "Get with the program": Pharmaceutical marketing, symptom checklists and self-diagnosis. *Social Science & Medicine, 73*, 825–832.

Effing, T. W., Kerstjens, H., van der Valk, P., Zielhuis, G. A., & van der Palen, J. (2009). The (cost)-effectivenes of self-treatment of exacerbations on the severity of exacerbations in COPD patients: The COPE study. *Thorax, 64*, 956–962.

Ehrlich-Jones, L., Lee, J., Semanik, P., Cox, C., Dunlop, D., & Chang, R. W. (2011). Relationship between beliefs, motivation and worries about physical activity and physical activity participation in persons with rheumatoid arthritis. *Arthritis Care & Research (Hoboken), 63*, 1700–1705.

Emmons, K. K. (2010). *Black dogs and blue words.* Piscataway, NJ: Rutgers University Press.

Estes, T. S. (2011). Moving towards effective chronic illness management: Asthma as an exemplar. *Chronic Respiratory Disease, 8*, 163–170.

Factor, R., Kawachi, I., & Williams, D. R. (2011). Understanding high risk behavior among non-dominant minorities: a social resistance framework. *Social Science & Medicine, 73*, 1292–1301.

Faden, R. R., Beauchamp, T. L., & Kass, N. E. (2011). Learning health care systems and justice. *The Hastings Center Report, 41*, 3.

Faden, R. R., & Powers, M. (2011). A social justice framework for health and science policy. *Cambridge Quarterly of Healthcare Ethics, 20*, 596–604.

Farrell, C., Molassiotis, A., Beaver, K., Heaven, C. (2011). Exploring the scope of oncologist specialist nurses' practice in the UK. *European Journal of Oncology Nursing, 15*, 160–166.

Feldman, S., & Gellert, P. (2006). The seductive quality of central human capabilities: Sociological insights into Nussbaum and Sen's disagreement. *Economy and Society, 35*, 423–452.

Fisher, E. B., Earp, J., Maman, S., & Zolotor, A. (2010). Cross-cultural and international adaptation of peer support for diabetes management. *Family Practice, 27*(Suppl. 1), 6–16.

Fiske, S. T. (2011). *Envy up, scorn down: How status divides us.* New York, NY: Russell Sage Foundation.

Fitzner, K., Dietz, D. A., & Moy, E. (2011). How innovative treatment models and data use are improving diabetes care among African American adults. *Population Health Management, 14*, 143–155.

Fitzner, K., Greenwood, D., Payne, H., Thomson, J., Vukovljak, L., McCulloch, A., & Specker, J. E. (2008). An assessment of patient education and self-management in diabetes disease management—two case studies. *Population Health Management, 11*, 329–340.

Funnell, M. M. (2010). Peer-based behavioural strategies to improve chronic disease self-management and clinical outcomes: Evidence, logistics, evaluation considerations and needs for future research. *Family Practice, 27*(Suppl. 1), 17–22.

Furler, J., Walker, C., Blackberry, I., Dunning, T., Sulaiman, N., Dunbar, J., … Young, D. (2008). The emotional context of self-management in chronic illness: a qualitative study of the role of health professional support in the self-management of type 2 diabetes. *BMC Health Services Research, 8*, 214.

Gage, E. A., Pailler, M., Zevon, M. A., Ch'ng, J., Groman, A., Kelly, M., … Gruber, M. (2011). Structuring survivorship care: Discipline-specific clinical perspectives. *Journal of Cancer Survivorship, 5*, 217–225.

Gallacher, K., May, C. P., Montori, V. M., & Mair, F. S. (2011). Understanding patients' experiences of treatment burden in chronic heart failure using normalization process theory. *Annals of Family Medicine, 9*, 235–243.

Gallagher, M., Worth, A., Cunningham-Burley, S., & Sheikh, A. (2011). Epinephrine auto-injector use in adolescents at risk of anaphylaxis:

A qualitative study in Scotland, UK. *Clinical and Experimental Allergy, 41,* 869–877.

Gallant, M. P., Spitze, G., & Grove, J. G. (2010). Chronic illness self-care and the family lives of older adults: A synthetic review across four ethnic groups. *Journal of Cross Cultural Gerontology, 25,* 21–43.

Geneau, R., Stuckler, D., Stachenko, S., McKee, M., Ebrahim, S., Basu, S., ... Beaglehole, R. (2010). Raising the priority of preventing chronic diseases: A political process. *Lancet, 376,* 1689–1698.

Ghahari, S., Packer, T. L., & Passmore, A. E. (2009). Development, standardization and pilot testing of an online fatigue self-management program. *Disability and Rehabilitation, 31,* 1762–1772.

Given, B. A. (2010). Symptom management in oncology care—Where are we? *European Journal of Oncology Nursing, 14,* 357–358.

Glasgow, R. E., Wagner, E. H., Schaefer, J., Mahoney, L. D., Reid, R. J., & Greene, S. M. (2005). Development and validation of the Patient Assessment of Chronic Illness Care (PACIC). *Medical Care, 43*(5), 436–444.

Glasgow, R. E., Whitesides, H., Nelson, C. C., & King, D. K. (2005). Use of the Patient Assessment of Chronic Illness Care (PACIC) with diabetic patients: Relationship to patient characteristics, receipt of care, and self-management. *Diabetes Care, 28*(11), 2655–2661.

Glenn, E. N. (2010). *Forced to care: Coercion and caregiving in America.* Cambridge, MA: Harvard University Press.

Goldman, D., & Smith, J. P. (2011). The increasing value of education to health. *Social Science & Medicine, 72,* 1728–1737.

Greene, J. A., Choudhry, N. K., Kilabuk, E., & Shrank, W. H. (2011). Online social networking by patients with diabetes: A qualitative evaluation of communication with facebook. *Journal of General Internal Medicine, 26,* 287–292.

Greenhalgh, T., Collard, A., Campbell-Richards, D., Vijayaraghavan, S., Malik, F., Morris, J., & Claydon, A. (2011). Storylines of self-management: Narratives of people with diabetes from a multiethnic inner city population. *Journal of Health Services Research Policy, 16,* 37–43.

Groessl, E. J., Weingart, K. R., Stepnowsky, C. J., Gifford, A. L., Asch, S. M., & Ho, S. B. (2011). The hepatitis self-management programme: A randomized controlled trial. *Journal of Viral Hepatitis, 18,* 358–368.

Greenop, D, Glenn, S, Ledson, M, Walshaw, M, *Self-care and cystic fibrosis: a review of research with adults, Health and Social Care in the Community* 18:653–661, 2010.

Gutmann, A. (2011). The ethics of synthetic biology: Guiding principles for emerging technologies. *Hastings Center Report, 41*(4), 17–22.

Hamann, J., Mendel, R., Buhner, M., Kissling, W., Cohen, R., Knipfer, E., & Eckstein, H. H. (in press). How should patients behave to facilitate shared decision making—the doctor's view. *Health Expect.*

Hamnes, B., Hauge, M. I., Kjeken, I., & Hagen, K. B. (2011). "I have come here to learn how to cope with my illness, not to be cured": A qualitative study of patient expectations prior to a one-week self-management programme. *Musculoskeletal Care, 9*, 200–210.

Hardisty, A. R., Peirce, S. C., Preece, A., Bolton, C. E., Conley, E. C., Gray, W. A., ... Elwyn, G. (2011). Bridging two translation gaps: A new informatics research agenda for telemonitoring of chronic disease. *International Journal of Medical Informatics, 80*, 734–744.

Healthy People 2010. Washington, DC: Department of Health and Human Services.

Heeson, C., Solari, A., Giordano, A., Kasper, J., & Kopke, S. (2011). Decisions on multiple sclerosis immune therapy: New treatment complexities urge patient engagement. *Journal of the Neurological Sciences, 306*, 192–197.

Heinemann, L. (2010). Quality of glucose measurement with blood glucose meters at the point-of-care: Relevance of interfering factors. *Diabetes Technology & Therapeutics, 12*, 847–857.

Heinrich, E., Candel, M. J., Schaper, N. C., & de Vries, N. K. (2010). Effect evaluation of a motivational interviewing based counseling strategy in diabetes care. *Diabetes Research and Clinical Practice, 90*, 270–278.

Heisler, M. (2010). Different models to mobilize peer support to improve diabetes self-management and clinical outcomes: Evidence, logistics, evaluation considerations and needs for future research. *Family Practice, 27*(Suppl. 1), 23–32.

Hekler, E. B., Lambert, J., Leventhal, E., Leventhal, H., Jahn, E., & Contrada, R. J. (2008). Commonsense illness beliefs, adherence behaviors, and hypertension control among African Americans. *Journal of Behavioral Medicine, 31*, 391–400.

Heneghan, C., Ward, A., Perera, R., & The Self-Monitoring Trialist Collaboration. (2012). Self-monitoring of oral anticoagulation: Systemic review and meta-analysis of individual patient data. *Lancet, 379*, 322–334.

Hewlett, S., Sanderson, T., May, J., Alten, R., Bingham, C. O., 3rd., Cross, M., ... Bartlett, S. J. (2012). I'm hurting, I want to kill myself: Rheumatoid arthritis flare is more than a high joint count—An international patient perspective on flare where medical help is sought. *Rheumatology, 51,* 69–76.

Hibbard, J. H. (2005). Development and testing of a short-form of the Patient Activation Measure. *Health Services Research, 40,* 1918–1930.

Hibbard, J. H., Greene, J., & Tusler, M. (2009). Improving the outcomes of disease management by tailoring care to the patient's level of activation. *American Journal of Managed Care, 15*(6), 353–360.

Hibbard, J. H., Mahoney, E. R., Stock, R., & Tusler, M. (2005). Development and testing of a short form of the patient activation measure. *Health Services Research, 40*(6 Pt 1), 1918–1930.

Hibbard, J. H., Mahoney, E. R., Stock, R., & Tusler, M. (2007). Do increases in patient activation result in improved self-management behaviors? *Health Services Research, 42*(4), 1443–1463.

Hibbard, J. H., Stockard, J., Mahoney, E. R., & Tusler, M. (2004). Development of the Patient Activation Measure (PAM): Conceptualizing and measuring activation in patients and consumers. *Health Services Research, 39*(4 Pt 1), 1005–1026.

Hicks, D. (2011). *Dignity: The essential role it plays in resolving conflict.* New Haven, CT: Yale University Press.

Holm, S., & Davies, M. (2009). Ethical issues around evidence-based patient choice and shared decision-making. In A. Edwards & G. Elwyn (Eds.), *Shared decision-making in health care* (2nd ed.). New York, NY: Oxford University Press.

Holroyd-Leduc, J. M., Straus, S., Thorpe, K., Davis, D. A., Schmaltz, H., & Tannenbaum, C. (2011). Translation of evidence into a self-management tool for use by women with urinary incontinence. *Age Ageing, 40,* 227–233.

Hopper, K. (2007). Rethinking social recovery in schizophrenia: What a capabilities approach might offer. *Social Science & Medicine, 65,* 868–879.

Hurley, M. V., Walsh, N., Bhavnani, V., Britten, N., & Stevenson, F. (2010). Health beliefs before and after participation in an exercise-based rehabilitation programme for chronic knee pain: Doing is believing. *BMC Musculoskelet Disorders, 11,* 31.

Ingles, S. C., Clark, R. A., McAlister, F. A., Stewart, S., & Cleland, J. G. (2011). Which components of heart failure programmes are effective? A systematic review and meta-analysis of the outcome of structured telephone support or telemonitoring as the primary component of chronic heart failure management in 8323 patients: Abridged Cochrane Review. *European Journal of Heart Failure, 13,* 1028–1040.

Ioannidis, J. P. (2009). Adverse events in randomized trials: Neglected, restricted, distorted, and silenced. *Archives of Internal Medicine, 169,* 1737–1739.

Iversen, M. D., Hammond, A., & Betteridge, N. (2010). Self-management of rheumatic diseases: state of the art and future perspectives. *Annals of the Rheumatic Diseases, 69,* 955–963.

Jacobson, N. (2009). Dignity violation in health care. *Qualitative Health Research, 19,* 1536–1547.

James, J. (2010). Diabetes specialist nursing in the UK: The judgement call? A review of existing literature. *Practical Diabetes, 27,* 248–253.

Jaremo, P., & Arman, M. (2011). Causes of illness—constraining and facilitating beliefs. *International Journal of Nursing Practice, 17,* 370–379.

Jennings, B. (2011). Bioethics between two worlds: The politics of ethics in Central Europe. In C. Myser (Ed.), *Bioethics around the globe.* New York, NY: Oxford University Press.

Joanna Briggs Institute. (2009). Effectiveness of interventions using empowerment concept for patients with chronic disease: A systematic review. *Journal of Advanced Nursing, 7,* 1446–1447.

John, H., Carroll, D., & Kitas, G. D. (2011). Cardiovascular education for people with rheumatoid arthritis: What can existing patient education programmes teach us? *Rheumatology (Oxford), 50,* 1751–1759.

Jonsson, P. D. (2010). *Living with bipolar disorder.* Sweden: University of Gothenburg. Retrieved from http://gupea.ub.gu.se/bitstream/2077/22944/2/gupea_2077_22944_2.pdf

Jordan, J. E., Osborne, R. H., & Buchbinder, R. (2011). Critical appraisal of health literacy indices revealed variable underlying constructs, narrow content and psychometric weaknesses. *Journal of Clinical Epidemiology, 64,* 366–379.

Joseph-Williams, N., Edwards, A., & Elwyn, G. (2011). The importance and complexity of regret in the measurement of "good" decisions: A systematic review and a content analysis of existing assessment instruments. *Health Expectations, 14,* 59–83.

Kaplan, R. S., & Porter, M. E. (2011). How to solve the cost crisis in health care. *Harvard Business Review, 89*(9), 46–61.

Kaptein, A. D., & Broadbent, E. (2007). Illness cognition assessment. In S. Ayers, A. Baum, C. McManus, S. Newman, K. Wallston, J. Weinman, & R. West (Eds.), *Cambridge handbook of psychology, health and medicine* (2nd ed.). Cambridge, UK: Cambridge University Press.

Kaya, Z., Erkan, F., Ozkan, M., Ozkan, S., Kocamin, N., Ertekin, B. A., & Direk, N. (2009). Self-management plans for asthma control and predictors of patient compliance. *The Journal of Asthma, 46,* 270–275.

Kleinman, A. (2007). *What really matters: Living a moral life amidst uncertainty and danger.* New York, NY: Oxford University Press.

Kleinman, A., & Hall-Clifford, R. (2010). Chronicity—time, space and culture. In L. Manderson & C. Smith-Morris (Eds.), *Chronic conditions, fluid states: Chronicity and the anthropology of illness.* New Brunswick, NJ: Rutgers University Press.

Klonoff, D. C., Cembrowski, G., Charpentier, G., Gabbay, R., Nicolucci, A., & Vigersky, R. (2011). Consensus report: the current role of self-monitoring of blood glucose in non-insulin-treated type 2 diabetes. *Journal of Diabetes Science and Technology, 5,* 1529–1548.

Kneck, A., Klang, B., & Faberberg, I. (2011). Learning to live with illness: Experiences of persons with recent diagnosis of diabetes mellitus. *Scandinavian Journal of Caring Sciences, 25,* 558–566.

Kolb, H., Kempf, K., Martin, S., Stumvoll, M., & Landgraf, R. (2010). On what evidence-base do we recommend self-monitoring of blood glucose? *Diabetes Research and Clinical Practice, 87,* 150–156.

Kovacs, J. (2010). The transformation of (bio)ethics expertise in a world of ethical pluralism. *Journal of Medical Ethics, 36,* 767–770.

Kroenke, K., Bair, M. J., Damush, T. M., Wu, J., Hoke, S., Sutherland, J., & Tu, W. (2009). Optimized antidepressant therapy and pain self-management in primary care patients with depression and musculoskeletal pain. *JAMA, 301,* 2099–2110.

Kvedar, J. C., Nesbitt, T., Kvedar, J. G., & Darkins, A. (2011). E-patient connectivity and the near term future. *Journal of General Internal Medicine, 26*(Suppl. 2), 636–638.

LaChapelle, D. L., Lavoie, S., & Boudreau, A. (2008). The meaning and process of pain acceptance. Perceptions of women living with arthritis and fibromyalgia. *Pain Research & Management, 13,* 201–210.

Lagger, G., Pataky, Z., & Golay, A. (2010). Efficacy of therapeutic patient education in chronic diseases and obesity. *Patient Education and Counseling, 79,* 283–286.

Lee, C. S., Moser, D. K., Lennie, T. A., & Riegßel, B. (2011). Event-free survival in adults with heart failure who engage in self-care management. *Heart Lung, 40,* 12–20.

Leino-Kilpi, H. (2011, February). *Outcome measures in patient education and learning—where is the knowledge basis?* Paper presented at State of

Science of Patient Education and Learning Conference, University of Gothenberg, Sweden.

Leventhal, H., Yael, B., & Shafer, C. (2007). Lay beliefs about heath and illness. In S. Ayers, A. Baum, C. McManus, S. Newman, K. Wallston, J. Weinman, & R. West (Eds.), *Cambridge handbook of psychology, health and medicine* (2nd ed.). Cambridge, UK: Cambridge University Press.

Liang, S.-Y., Yates, P., Edwards, H., & Tsay, S.-L. (2012). Opioid-taking self-efficacy among Taiwanese outpatients with cancer. *Supportive Care in Cancer, 20,* 199–206.

Light, B., & McGrath, K. (2010). Ethics and social networking sites: A disclosive analysis of Facebook. *Information Technology & People, 23,* 290–311.

Lippa, K. D., Klein, H. A., & Shalin, V. L. (2008). Everyday expertise: Cognitive demands in diabetes self-management. *Human Factors, 50,* 112–120.

Loriq, K. R., Sobel, D. S. et al, Evidence suggesting that a chronic disease self-management program can improve health status while reducing hospitalization, *Medical Care* 1999 37: 5–14

Louw, A., Diener, I., Butler, D. S., & Puentedura, E. J. (2011). The effect of neuroscience education on pain, disability, anxiety and stress in chronic musculoskeletal pain. *Archives of Physical Medicine and Rehabilitation, 92,* 2041–2056.

Lundahl, B. W., Kunz, C., Brownell, C., Tollefson, D., & Burke, B. L. (2010). A meta-analysis of motivational interviewing: Twenty-five years of empirical studies. *Research on Social Work Practice, 20,* 137–160.

Lutfey, K. E., & Freese, J. (2007). Ambiguities of chronic illness management and challenges to the medical error paradigm. *Social Science & Medicine, 64,* 314–325.

Lynch, C. P., & Egede, L. E. (2011). Optimizing diabetes self-care in low literacy and minority populations—problem-solving, empowerment, peer support and technology-based approaches. *Journal of General Internal Medicine, 26,* 953–955.

Malmusi, D., Artazcoz, L., Benach, J., & Borrell, C. (2011). Perception or real illness? How chronic conditions contribute to gender inequalities in self-rated health. *European Journal of Pain.* Advance online publication.

Manning, S. (2011). Bridging the gap between hospital and home: a new model of care for reducing readmission rates in chronic heart failure. *The Journal of Cardiovascular Nursing, 26,* 368–376.

Martinez, W., Carter, J. S., & Legato, L. J. (2011). Social competence in children with chronic illness: A meta-analytic review. *Journal of Pediatric Psychology, 36,* 878–870.

Martino, S. (2011). Motivational interviewing to engage patients in chronic kidney disease management. *Blood Purification, 31*, 77–81.

Mathar, T. (2011). Managing health(-care systems) using information health technologies. *Health Care Analysis, 19*, 180–191.

Mausbach, B. T., Moore, R., Bowie, C., Cardenas, V., & Patterson, T. L. (2009). A review of instruments for measuring functional recovery in those diagnosed with psychosis. *Schizophrenia Bulletin, 35*, 307–318.

May, S. (2010). Self-management of chronic low back pain and osteoarthritis. Nature Reviews. *Rheumatology, 6*, 199–209.

McAteer, A., Elliott, A. M., & Hannaford, P. C. (2011). Ascertaining the size of the symptom iceberg in a UK-wide community-based survey. *The British Journal of General Practice, 61*(582), 12–17.

McCabe, P. J., Schumacher, K., & Barnason, S. A. (2011). Living with atrial fibrillation: A qualitative study. *The Journal of Cardiovascular Nursing, 26*, 336–344.

McCorkle, R., Ercolano, E., Lazenby, M., Schulman-Green, D., Schilling, L. S., Lorig, K., & Wagner, E. H. (2011). Self-management: Enabling and empowering patients living with cancer as a chronic illness. *CA: A Cancer Journal for Clinicians, 61*, 50–62.

McDonald, V. M., Vertigan, A. E., & Gibson, P. G. (2011). How to set up a severe asthma service. *Respirology, 16*, 900–911.

McManus, R. J., Mant, J., Bray, E. P., Holder, R., Jones, M. I., Greenfield, S., … Hobbs, F. D. (2010). Telemonitoring and self-management in the control of hypertension (TASMINH 2): A randomized controlled trial. *Lancet, 376*, 163–172.

Michalak, E., Livingston, J. D., Hole, R., Suto, M., Hale, S., & Haddock, C. (2011). "It's something that I manage but it is not who I am": Reflections on internalized stigma in individuals with bipolar disorder. *Chronic Illness, 7*, 209–224.

Miles, A., & Loughlin, M. (2011). Models in the balance: evidence-based medicine versus evidence-informed individualized care. *Journal of Evaluation in Clinical Practice, 17*, 531–536.

Miles, C. L., Pincus, T., Carnes, D., Taylor, S. J., & Underwood, M. (2011). Measuring pain self-efficacy. *Clinical Journal of Pain, 27*(5), 461–470.

Millett, C., Netuveli, G., Saxena, S., & Majeed, A. (2009). Impact of pay for performance on ethnic disparities in intermediate outcomes for diabetes: A longitudinal study. *Diabetes Care, 32*, 404–409.

Minet, L., Moller, S., Vach, W., Wagner, L., & Henriksen, J. E. (2010). Mediating the effect of self-care management intervention in type 2 diabetes: A meta-analysis of 47 randomised controlled trials. *Patient Education and Counseling, 80,* 29–41.

Minet, L. K. R., Lonvig, E. M., Henriksen, J. E., & Wagner, L. (2011). The experience of living with diabetes following a self-management program based on motivational interviewing. *Qualitative Health Research, 21,* 1115–1126.

Miranda, V., Fede, A., Nobuo, M., Ayres, V., Giglio, A., Miranda, M., & Riechelmann, R. P. (2011). Adverse drug reactions and drug interactions as causes of hospital admissions in oncology. *Journal of Pain and Symptom Management, 42,* 342–353.

Mosen, D. M., Schmittdiel, J., Hibbard, J., Sobel, D., Remmers, C., & Bellows, J. (2007). Is patient activation associated with outcomes of care for adults with chronic conditions? *Journal of Ambulatory Care Management, 30*(1), 21–29.

Mullis, R., & Hay, E. M. (2010). Goal scaling for low back pain in primary care: Development of a semi-structured interview incorporating minimal important change. *Journal of Evaluation in Clinical Practice, 16,* 1209–1214.

Muntner, P., Woodward, M., Carson, A. P., Judd, S. E., Levitan, E. B., Mann, D. M., ... Warnock, D. G. (2011). Development and validation of a self-assessment tool for albuminuria: Results from the Reasons for Geographic and Racial Differences in Stroke (REGARDS) Study. *American Journal of Kidney Diseases, 58,* 196–205.

Murad, M. H., Shah, N. D., Van Houten, H. K., Zeigenfuss, J. Y., Deming, J. R., Beebe, T. J., ... Montori, V. M. (2011). Individuals with diabetes preferred that future trials use patient-important outcomes and provide pragmatic inferences. *Journal of Clinical Epidemiology, 64,* 743–748.

Murray, E. T., Jennings, I., Kitchen, D., Kitchen, S., & Fitzmaurice, D. A. (2007). Quality assurance for oral anticoagulation self-management: A cluster randomized trial. *Journal of Thrombosis and Haemostasis, 6,* 464–469.

Nicolaidis, C. (2011). Police officer, deal-maker, or health care provider? Moving to a patient-centered framework for chronic opioid management. *Pain Medicine, 12,* 890–897.

Nielsen, A. B., Gannik, D., Siersma, V., & Olivarius Nde, F. (2011). The relationship between HbA1c level, symptoms and self-rated health in type 2 diabetic patients. *Scandinavian Journal of Primary Health Care, 29,* 157–164.

Nissen, M. J., Tsai, M. L., Blaes, A. H., & Swenson, K. K. (in press). Breast and colorectal cancer survivors' knowledge about their diagnosis and treatment. *Journal of Cancer Survivorship.*

Norweg, A., Ni, P., Garshick, E., O'Connor, G., Wilke, K, & Jette, A. M. (2011). A multidimensional computer adaptive test approach to dyspnea assessment. *Archives of Physical Medicine and Rehabilitation, 92,* 1561–1569.

Nowak, R. (2008, November 8). The online doctor will see you now. *New Scientist, 200,* 24–25.

Nussbaum, M. C. (2000). *Women and human development: The capabilities approach.* Cambridge, UK: University Press.

Nussbaum, M. C. (2009). Dignity and political entitlements. In E. D. Pellegrino, A. Schulman, & T. W. Merrill (Eds.), *Human dignity and bioethics.* Notre Dame, IN: University Press.

Nussbaum, M. C. (2011). *Creating capabilities: The human development approach.* Cambridge, MA: Harvard University Press.

Ogawa, M., Miyamoto, Y., & Kawakami, N. (2011). Factors associated with glycemic control and diabetes self-care among outpatients with schizophrenia and type 2 diabetes. *Archives of Psychiatric Nursing, 25,* 63–73.

Ohnsorge, K., & Widdershoven, G. (2011). Monological versus dialogical consciousness—two epistomological views on the use of theory in clinical ethical practice. *Bioethics, 25,* 361–369.

Or, C. K., Karsh, B. T., Severtson, D. J., Burke, L. J., Brown, R. L., & Brennan, P. F. (2011). Factors affecting home care patients' acceptance of a web-based interactive self-management technology. *Journal of the American Medical Informatics Association 18,* 51–59.

Ozura, A., Erdberg, P., & Sega, S. (2010). Personality characteristics of multiple sclerosis patients: A rorschach investigation. *Clinical Neurology and Neurosurgery, 112,* 629–632.

Pampel, F. C., Krueger, P. M., & Denney, J. T. (2010). Socioeconomic disparities in health behaviors. *Annual Review of Sociology, 36,* 349–370.

Parajes, F. (2008). Motivational role of self-efficacy beliefs in self-regulated learning. In D. H. Schunk & B. J. Zimmerman (Eds.), *Motivation and self-regulated learning.* New York, NY: Lawrence Erlbaum and Associates.

Parchman, M. L., Zeber, J. E., Romero, R. R., & Pugh, J. A. (2007). Risk of coronary artery disease in type 2 diabetes and the delivery of care consistent with the chronic care model in primary care settings. *Medical Care, 45*(12), 1129–1134.

Parekh, A. K., Goodman, R. A., Gordon, C., Koh, H. K., & HHS Interagency Workgroup on Chronic Conditions. (2011). Managing multiple chronic conditions: A strategic framework for improving health outcomes and quality of life. *Public Health Reports, 126,* 460–471.

Parens, E., & Johnston, J. (2009). Facts, values and attention-deficit hyperactivity disorder (ADHD): An update on the controversies. *Child and Adolescent Psychiatry and Mental Health, 3,* 1.

Partridge, E. E., Mayer-Davis, E. J., Sacco, R. L., & Balch, A. J. (2011). Creating a 21st century global health agenda: The General Assembly of the United Nations high level meeting on non-communicable diseases. *CA: A Cancer Journal for Clinicians, 61,* 209–211.

Patel, N. K., & Parchman, M. L. (2011). The chronic care model and exercise discussions during primary care diabetes encounters. *Journal of the American Board of Family Medicine, 24*(1), 26–32.

Peel, E., Douglas, M., & Lawton, J. (2007). Self-monitoring of blood glucose in type 2 diabetes: Longitudinal qualitative study of patients' perspectives. *British Medical Journal, 335,* 493–498.

Penfornis, A., Personeni, E., & Borot, S. (2011). Evolution of devices in diabetes management. *Diabetes Technology & Therapeutics, 13*(Suppl. 1), S93–S102.

Perez, X., Wisnivesky, J. P., Lurslurchachai, L., Kleinman, L. C., & Kronish, I. M. (2012). Barriers to adherence to COPD guidelines among primary care providers. *Respiratory Medicine, 106,* 374–381.

Peters, R. M., Aroian, K. J., & Flack, J. M. Western (2006). African American culture and hypertension prevention. *Journal of Nursing Research, 28,* 831–863.

Petkov, J., Harvey, P., & Battersby, M. (2010). The internal consistency and construct validity of the partners in health scale: Validation of a patient rated chronic condition self-management measure. *Quality of Life Research, 19,* 1079–1085.

Petrie, K. J., Cameron, L. D., Ellis, C. J., Buick, D., & Weinman, J. (2002). Changing illness perceptions after myocardial infarction: An early intervention randomized controlled trial. *Psychosomatic Medicine, 64,* 580–586.

Piering, K., Arnon, R., Miloh, T. A., Florman, S., Kerkar, N., & Annunziato, R. A. (2011). Developmental and disease-related influence on self-management and acquisition among pediatric liver transplant recipients. *Pediatric Transplantation, 15,* 819–826.

Pink, J., Pink, K., & Elwyn, G. (2009). Measuring patient knowledge of asthma: A systematic review of outcome measures. *The Journal of Asthma, 46,* 980–987.

Piot, P., & Ebrahim, S. (2010). Prevention and control of chronic diseases. *BMJ, 341,* c4865.

Porter, S., O'Halloran, P., & Morrow, E. (2011). Bringing values back into evidence-based nursing. *ANS Advances in Nursing Science, 34,* 106–118.

Porz, R., Landeweer, E., & Widdershoven, G. (2011). Theory and practice of clinical ethics support services: Narrative and hermeneutical perspectives. *Bioethics, 25,* 354–360.

Powers, B. J., Olsen, M. K., Smith, V. A., Woolson, R. F., Bosworth, H. B., & Oddone, E. Z. (2011). Measuring blood pressure for decision making and quality reporting: Where and how many measures? *Annals of Internal Medicine, 154,* 781–788.

Press, V. G., Arora, V. M., Shah, L. M., Lewis, S. L., Ivy, K., Charbeneau, J., ... Krishnan, J. A. (2011). Misuse of respiratory inhalers in hospitalized patients with asthma and COPD. *Journal of General Internal Medicine, 26,* 635–642.

Pring, R. (2004). *Philosophy of educational research* (2nd ed.). London, England: Continuum.

Qamar, M., Bender, F., Rault, R., & Piraino, B. (2009). The United States' perspectives on home dialysis. *Advances in Chronic Kidney Disease, 16,* 189–197.

Redman, B. K. (2007). Responsibility for control: Ethics of patient preparation for self-management of chronic disease. *Bioethics, 21,* 243–250.

Redman, B. K. (2009). Patient adherence or patient self-management in transplantation: An ethical analysis. *Progress in Transplantation, 19,* 90–94.

Regnier-Denois, V., Rousset-Guarato, V., Nourissat, A., Bourmaud, A., & Chauvin, F. (2009). Contribution of a preliminary socio-anthropological survey to the development of a therapeutic patient education programme for patients receiving oral chemotherapy. *Therapeutic Patient Education, 2,* S101–S107.

Reid, M. C., Bennett, D. A., Chen, W. G., Eldadah, B. A., Farrar, J. T., Ferrell, B., ... Zacharoff, K. L. (2011). Improving the pharmacologic management of pain in older adults: Identifying the research gaps and methods to address them. *Pain Medicine, 12,* 1336–1357.

Riegel, B., Lee, C. S., Albert, N., Lennie, T., Chung, M., Song, E. K., ... Moser, D. K. (2011). From novice to expert: Confidence and activity status determine heart failure self-care performance. *Nursing Research, 60,* 132–138.

Riegel, B., Moser, D. K., Anker, S. D., Appel, L. J., Dunbar, S. B., Grady, K. L., ... Whellan, D. J. (2009). State of the science: Promoting self-care in persons with heart failure: A scientific statement from the American Heart Association. *Circulation, 120,* 1141–1163.

Ring, N., Jepson, R., Hoskins, G., Wilson, C., Pinnock, H., Sheikh, A., & Wyke, S. (2011). Understanding what helps or hinders action plan use: A systematic review and synthesis of the qualitative literature. *Patient Education and Counseling, 85,* e131–e143.

Ritzema, J., Troughton, R., Melton, I., Crozier, I., Doughty, R., Krum, H., ... Hemodynamically Guided Home Self-Therapy in Severe Heart Failure Patients (HOMEOSTASIS) Study Group. (2010). Physician-directed patient self-management of left atrial pressure in advanced chronic heart failure. *Circulation, 121,* 1086–1095.

Roark, R. F., Shah, B. R., Udayakumar, K., & Peterson, E. D. (2011). The need for transformative innovation in hypertension management. *American Heart Journal, 162,* 405–411.

Robeyns, I. (2005). The capability approach: A theoretical survey. *Journal of Human Development, 6,* 93–114.

Rogers, A., Bury, M., & Kennedy, A. (2009). Rationality, rhetoric, and religiosity in health care: The case of England's Expert Patients Programme. *International Journal of Health Services, 39,* 725–747.

Rogers, A., Kirk, S., Gately, C., May, C. R., & Finch, T. (2011). Established users and the making of telecare work in long term condition management: Implications for health policy. *Social Science & Medicine, 72,* 1077–1084.

Rollnick, S., Butler, C. C., Kinnersley, P., Gregory, J., & Mash, B. (2010). Motivational interviewing. *British Medical Journal, 340,* 1242–1245.

Rosemann, T., Laux, G., Droesemeyer, S., Gensichen, J., & Szecsenyi, J. (2007). Evaluation of a culturally adapted German version of the Patient Assessment of Chronic Illness Care (PACIC 5A) questionnaire in a sample of osteoarthritis patients. *Journal of Evaluation in Clinical Practice, 13*(5), 806–813.

Rosland, A., & Piette, J. D. (2010). Emerging models for mobilizing family support for chronic disease management: A structured review. *Chronic Illness, 6,* 7–21.

Rosser, B. A., & Eccleston, C. (2011). Smartphone applications for pain management. *Journal of Telemedicine and Telecare, 17,* 308–312.

Roter, D. L. (2011). Oral literacy demand of health care communication: Challenges and solutions. *Nursing Outlook, 59,* 79–84.

Rovner, B. W., Casten, R. J., Hegel, M. T., Massof, R. W., Leiby, B. E., & Tasman, W. S. (2011). Improving function in age-related macular degeneration: Design and methods of a randomized clinical trial. *Contemporary Clinical Trials, 32,* 196–203.

Ryan, F., O'Shea, S., & Byrne, S. (2010). The "carry-over" effects of patient self-testing: Positive effects on usual care management by an antico-agulation management service. *Thrombosis Research, 126,* e345–e348.

Saarni, S. I., Braunack-Mayer, A., Hofmann, B., & van der Wilt, G. J. (2011). Different methods for ethical analysis in health technology assessment: An empirical study. *International Journal of Technology Assessment in Health Care, 27,* 305–312.

Sadof, M., & Kaslovsky, R. (2011). Adolescent asthma: A developmental approach. *Current Opinion in Pediatrics, 23,* 373–378.

Sajadi, K. P., & Goldman, H. B. (2011). Social networks lack useful content for incontinence. *Urology, 78,* 764–767.

Sanderson, T. C., Hewlett, S. E., Flurey, C., Dures, E., Richards, P., & Kirwan, J. R. (2011). The impact triad (severity, importance, self-management) as a method of enhancing measurement of personal life impact of rheumatic diseases. *Journal of Rheumatology, 38,* 191–194.

Sarkar, U., Handley, M. A., Gupta, R., Tang, A., Murphy, E., Seligman, H. K., . . . Schillinger, D. (2008). Use of an interactive, telephone-based self-management support program to identify adverse events among ambulatory diabetes patients. *Journal of General Internal Medicine, 23,* 459–465.

Schermer, M. (2009). Telecare and self-management: Opportunity to change the paradigm? *Journal of Medical Ethics, 35,* 688–691.

Schillinger, D. (2011). Supporting self management—a necessity in diabetes health care. *Patient Education and Counseling, 85,* 131–132.

Schmid-Buchi, S., Halfens, R., Dassen, T., & van den Borne, B. (2011). Psychosocial problems and needs of post-treatment patients with breast cancer and their relatives. *European Journal of Oncology Nursing, 15,* 260–266.

Schulman-Green, D., Bradley, E. H., Knobf, M. T., Prigerson, H., DiGiovanna, M. P., & McCorckle, R. (2011). Self-management and transition in women with advanced breast cancer. *Journal of Pain and Symptom Management, 42,* 517–525.

Scolaro, K. L., Lloyd, K. B., & Helms, K. L. (2008). Devices for home evaluation of women's health concerns. *American Journal of Health System Pharmacy, 65,* 299–314.

Scollan-Koliopoulos, M., Walker, E. A., Rapp, K. J., 3rd. (2011). Self-regulation theory and the multigenerational legacy of diabetes. *The Diabetes Educator, 37,* 669–679.

Seligman, H. K., & Schillinger, D. (2010). Hunger and socioeconomic disparities in chronic disease. *New England Journal of Medicine, 363,* 6–9.

Sen, A. (2009). *The idea of justice.* Cambridge, MA: Harvard University Press.

Shortus, T., Kemp, L., McKenzie, S., & Harris, M. (in press). Managing patient involvement: provider perspectives on diabetes decision making. *Health Expect.*

Shrivastava, A., Johnston, M., Shah, N., & Bureau, Y. (2010). Redefining outcome measures in schizophrenia: Integrating social and clinical parameters. *Current Opinion in Psychiatry, 23,* 120–126.

Sirotinin, S. V. & George, C. J. (2010). Computer-aided learning in insulin pump training. *Journal of Diabetes Science and Technology, 4,* 1022–1026.

Sklaroff, S. (2012). On our own: Why we who struggle to live with diabetes could use a helping hand. *Health Affairs, 31,* 236–239.

Skolasky, R. L., Green, A. F., Scharfstein, D., Boult, C., Reider, L., & Wegener, S. T. (2011). Psychometric properties of the patient activation measure among multimorbid older adults. *Health Services Research, 46*(2), 457–478.

Smith, J. R., Mugford, M., Holland, R., Noble, M. J., & Harrison, B. D. (2007). Psycho-educational interventions for adults with severe or difficult asthma: A systematic review. *The Journal of Asthma, 44,* 219–241.

Sonmez, A., Yilmaz, A., Uckaya, G., Kilic, S., Tapan, S., & Taslipinar, A. (2010). The accuracy of home glucose meters in hypoglycemia. *Diabetes Technology and Therapeutics, 12,* 619–626.

Soran, O. Z., Feldman, A. M., Pina, I. L., Lamas, G. A., Kelsey, S. F., Selzer, F., ... Lave, J. R. (2010). Cost of medical services in older patients with heart failure: Those receiving enhanced monitoring using a computer-based telephonic monitoring system compared with those in usual care: The heart failure home care trial. *Journal of Cardiac Failure, 16,* 859–866.

Stamm, T., van der Giesen, F., Thorstensson, C., Steen, E., Birrell, F., Bauernfeind, B., ... Kloppenburg, M. (2009). Patient perspective of hand osteoarthritis in relation to concepts covered by instruments measuring functioning: A qualitative European multicentre trial. *Annals of the Rheumatic Diseases, 68,* 1453–1460.

Standish, P., Smeyers, P., & Smith, R. (2007). *The therapy of education: Philosophy, happiness, and personal growth.* New York, NY: Palgrave Macmillan.

Starfield, B. (2011). Point: The changing nature of disease: Implications for health services. *Medical Care, 49,* 1971–1975.

Stein, P. D., Hull, R. D., Matta, F., & Willyerd, G. L. (2010). Modest response in translation to home management of deep vein thrombosis. *The American Journal of Medicine, 123,* 1107–1113.

Steurer-Stey, C., Frei, A., Schmid-Mohler, G., Malcolm-Kohler, S., Zoller, M., & Rosemann, T. (2010). Assessment of Chronic Illness Care with the German version of the ACIC in different primary care settings in Switzerland. *Health and Quality of Life Outcomes, 8,* 122.

Street, R. L., Jr., & Haidet, P. (2011). How well do doctors know their patients? Factors affecting physician understanding of patients' health beliefs. *Journal of General Internal Medicine, 26,* 21–27.

Suter, P., Hennessey, B., Florez, D., & Newton, S. W. (2011). The home-based chronic care model: redesigning home health for high quality care delivery. *Chronic Respiratory Disease, 8,* 43–52.

Suter, P., Suter, W. N., & Johnston, D. (2011). Theory-based telehealth and patient empowerment. *Population Health Management, 14,* 87–92.

Swindell, J. S., McGuire, A. L., & Halpern, S. D. (2010). Beneficent persuasion: techniques and ethical guidelines to improve patients' decisions. *Annals of Family Medicine, 8,* 260–264.

Szecsenyi, J., Rosemann, T., Joos, S., Peters-Klimm, F., & Miksch, A. (2008). German diabetes disease management programs are appropriate for restructuring care according to the Chronic Care Model. *Diabetes Care, 31,* 1150–1154.

Taggart, J., Chan, B., Jayasinghe, U. W., Christl, B., Proudfoot, J., Crookes, P., … Harris, M. F. (2011). Patients Assessment of Chronic Illness Care (PACIC) in two Australian studies: Structure and utility. *Journal of Evaluation in Clinical Practice, 17*(2), 215–221.

Taieb, O., Bricou, O., Baubet, T., Gabouland, V., Gal, B., Mouthon, L., … Moro, M. R. (2010). Patients' beliefs about the causes of systemic lupus erythematosus. *Rheumatology, 49,* 592–599.

Tang, T. S., Guadalupe, A. X., Cherrington, A., & Rana, G. (2011). A review of volunteer-based peer support interventions in diabetes. *Diabetes Spectrum, 24,* 85–98.

Thille, P. H., & Russell, G. M. (2010). Giving patients responsibility or fostering mutual response-ability: Family physicians' construction of effective chronic illness management. *Qualitative Health Research,* *20,* 1343–1352.

Thoits, P. A. (2011). Mechanisms linking social ties and support to physical and mental health. *Journal of Health and Social Behavior, 52,* 145–161.

Thompson, J. L., Sundt, T. M., Sarano, M. E., Santrach, P. J., & Schaff, H. V. (2008). In-patient international normalized ratio self-testing instruction after mechanical heart valve implantation. *The Annals of Thoracic Surgery, 85,* 2046–2050.

Thorne, S. (2006). Patient-provider communication in chronic illness: A health promotion window of opportunity. *Family & Community Health, 29*(Suppl. 1), 4S–11S.

Thorne, S. (2008). Chronic disease management: What is the concept? *Canadian Journal of Nursing Research, 40,* 7–14.

Thorne, S. E., Harris, S. R., Mahoney, K., Con, A., & McGuinness, L. (2004). The context of health care communication in chronic illness. *Patient Education and Counseling, 54,* 299–306.

Tranulis, C., Goff, D., Henderson, D. C., & Freudenreich, O. (2011). Becoming adherent to antipsychotics: A qualitative study of treatment-experienced schizophrenia patients. *Psychiatric Services, 62,* 888–892.

Trappenburg, J., Monninkhof, E. M., Bourbeau, J., Troosters, T., Schrijvers, A. J., Verheij, T. J., & Lammers, J. W. (2011). Effect of an action plan with ongoing support by a case manager on exacerbation-related outcomes in patients with COPD: A multicentre randomised controlled trial. *Thorax, 66,* 977–984.

Tugwell, P. S., Petersson, I. F., Boers, M., Gossec, L., Kirwan, J. R., Rader, T., ... Witter, J. P. (2011). Domain selection for patient-reported outcomes: Current activities and options for future methods. *Journal of Rheumatology, 38,* 1702–1710.

UnitedHealth, National Heart, Lung, and Blood Institute Centers of Excellence, Cerqueira, M. T., Cravioto, A., Dianis, N., Ghannem, H., Levitt, N., ... Smith, R. (2011). Global response to non-communicable disease. *British Medicine Journal, 342,* d3823.

Upton, J., Fletcher, M., Madoc-Sutton, H., Sheikh, A., Caress, A. L., & Walker, S. (2011). Shared decision making or paternalism in nursing consultations? A qualitative study of primary care asthma nurses' views on sharing decisions with patients regarding inhaler device selection. *Health Expect, 14,* 374–382.

Upton, J., Madoc-Sutton, H., Sheikh, A., Frank, T. L., Walker, S., & Fletcher, M. (2007). National survey on the roles and training of primary care respiratory nurses in the UK in 2006: are we making progress? *Primary Care Respiratory Journal, 16*, 284–290.

Vallerand, A. H., Templin, T., Hasenau, S. M., & Riley-Doucet, C. (2007). Factors that affect functional status in patients with cancer-related pain. *Pain, 132*, 82–90.

van Hooff, M. L., van der Merwe, J. D., O'Dowd, J., Pavlov, P. W., Spruit, M., de Kleuver, M., & van Limbeek, J. (2010). Daily functioning and self-management in patients with chronic low back pain after an intensive cognitive behavioral programme for pain management. *European Spine Journal, 19*, 1517–1526.

Vassilev, I. (2011). Social networks, social capital and chronic illness self-management: A realist review. *Chronic Illness, 7*, 60–86.

Vassilev, I., Rogers, A., Sanders, C., Kennedy, A., Blickem, C., Protheroe, J., … Morris, R. (2011). Social networks, social capital and chronic illness self-management: A realist review. *Chronic Illness, 7*, 60–86.

Veitch, K. (2010). The government of health care and the politics of patient empowerment: New labour and the NHS reform agenda in England. *Law and Policy, 32*, 313–331.

Voss, R., Gardner, R., Baier, R., Butterfield, K., Lehrman, S., & Gravenstein, S. (2011). The care transitions intervention: Translating from efficacy to effectiveness. *Archives of Internal Medicine, 171*, 1231–1237.

Walker, C. (2010). Ruptured identities: Leaving work because of chronic illness. *International Journal Health Services, 40*, 629–643.

Walker, H. A., & Chen, E. (2010). The impact of family asthma management on biology: A longitudinal investigation of youth with asthma. *Journal of Behavioral Medicine, 33*, 326–334.

Wallace, A., Carlson, J., Malone, R., Joyner, J., & DeWalt, D. (2010). The influence of literacy on patient-reported experiences of diabetes self-management support. *Nursing Research, 59*, 356–363.

Wamboldt, F. S., Bender, B. G., & Rankin, A. E. (2011). Adolescent decision making about use of inhaled asthma controller medication: Results from focus groups with participants from a prior longitudinal study. *Journal of Asthma, 48*, 741–750.

Warren-Findlow, J., Seymour, R. B., & Shenk, D. (2011). Intergenerational transmission of chronic illness self-care: Results from the caring for hypertension in African American families study. *Gerontologist, 51*, 64–75.

Washington, A. E., & Lipstein, S. H. (2011). The Patient-Centered Outcomes Research Institute—promoting better information, decisions and health. *New England Journal of Medicine, 365,* e31.

Wasserman, J. A., & Hinote, B. P. (2011). Chronic illness as incalculable risk: Scientific uncertainty and social transformations in medicine. *Social Theory and Health, 9,* 41–58.

Webb, S. (2011). Attacks on asthma. *Nature Biotechnology, 29,* 860–863.

Webel, A. R., & Okonsky, J. (2011). Psychometric properties of a symptom management self-efficacy scale for women living with HIV/AIDS. *Journal of Pain and Symptom Management, 41,* 549–557.

Weiner, T. (2011). The (un)managed self: Paradoxical forms of agency in self-management of bipolar disorder. *Culture, Medicine and Psychiatry, 35,* 448–483.

Weiss, M. E., Yakusheva, O., & Bobay, K. L. (2011). Quality and cost analysis of nurse staffing discharge preparation and post discharge utilization. *Health Services Research, 46,* 1473–1494.

Weitzman, E. R., Cole, E., Kaci, L., & Mandl, K. D. (2011). Social but safe? Quality and safety of diabetes-related online social networks. *Journal of the American Medical Informatics Association, 18,* 292–297.

Wennberg, J. E. (2010). *Tracking medicine: A researcher's quest to understand health care.* New York, NY: Oxford University Press.

Wensing, M., van Lieshout, J., Jung, H. P., Hermsen, J., & Rosemann, T. (2008). The Patients Assessment Chronic Illness Care (PACIC) questionnaire in The Netherlands: A validation study in rural general practice. [Validation Studies]. *BMC Health Services Research, 8,* 182.

White, R. O., 3rd., Osborn, C. Y., Gebretsadik, T., Kripalani, S., & Rothman, R. L. (2011). Development and validation of a Spanish diabetes-specific numeracy measure: DNT-15 Latino. *Diabetes Technology & Therapeutics, 13,* 893–898.

Wicks, P., Massagli, M., Frost, J., Brownstein, C., Okun, S., Vaughan, T., ... Heywood, J. (2010). Sharing health data for better outcomes on PatientsLikeMe. *Journal of Medical Internet Research, 12*(2), e19.

Williams, G., & Popay, J. (2006). Lay knowledge and the privilege of experience. In D. Kelleher, J. Gabe, & G. Williams (Eds.), *Challenging medicine* (2nd ed.). London, England: Routledge.

Williamson, C. (2008). The patient movement as an emancipation movement. *Health Expect, 11,* 102–112.

Wilson, P. M. (2008). The UK expert patients program: Lessons learned and implications for cancer survivors' self-care support programs. *Journal of Cancer Survivorship, 2,* 45–52.

Wilson, P. M., & Goodman, C. (2011). Evaluation of a modified chronic disease self-management programme for people with intellectual disabilities. *Journal of Nursing and Healthcare of Chronic Illness, 3,* 310–318.

Wirth, D. (2008). Incorporating self-testing into your practice. *Journal of Thrombosis and Thrombolysis, 25,* 12–13.

Wolff, J., & de-Shalit, A. (2007). *Disadvantage.* New York, NY: Oxford University Press.

Wright, J. A., Wallston, K. A., Elasy, T. A., Ikizler, T. A., & Cavanaugh, K. L. (2011). Development and results of a Kidney Disease Knowledge Survey given to patients with CKD. *American Journal of Kidney Diseases, 57,* 387–395.

Wu, F. L., Juang, J. H., & Yeh, M. C. (2011). The dilemma of diabetic patients living with hypoglycaemia. *Journal of Clinical Nursing, 20,* 2277–2285.

Wysocki, D. K., Nourjah, P., & Swartz, L. (2007). Bleeding complications with warfarin use: A prevalent adverse effect resulting in regulatory action. *Archives of Internal Medicine, 167,* 1414–1419.

Yamin, C. K., Emani, S., Williams, D. H., Lipsitz, S. R., Karson, A. S., Wald, J. S., & Bates, D. W. (2011). The digital divide in adoption and use of a personal health record. *Archives of Internal Medicine, 171,* 568–574.

Yen, L., Gillespie, J., Rn, Y. H., Kljakovic, M., Anne Brien, J., Jan, S., ... Usherwood, T. (2011). Health professionals, patients and chronic illness policy: A qualitative study. *Health Expectations, 14,* 10–20.

Young, H. N., Chan, M. R., Yevzlin, A. S., & Becker, B. N. (2011). The rationale, implementation and effect of the Medicare CKD education benefit. *American Journal of Kidney Diseases, 57,* 381–386.

Young, M. (2009). Basic capabilities, basic learning outcomes and thresholds of learning. *Journal of Human Development and Capabilities, 10,* 259–277.

Zafar, W., & Mojtabai, R. (2011). Chronic disease management for depression in US medical practices: Results from the Health Tracking Physician Survey. *Medical Care, 49,* 634–640.

Zoffmann, V., Harder, I., & Kirkevold, M. (2008). A person-centered communication and reflection model: shared decision-making in chronic care. *Qualitative Health Research, 18,* 670–685.

Index